Carbohydrate metabolism in plants

C. M. DUFFUS

*School of Agriculture, University of Edinburgh
and East of Scotland College of Agriculture*

J. H. DUFFUS

*Department of Brewing and Biological Sciences,
Heriot-Watt University, Edinburgh*

Longman
London and New York

Longman Group Limited
Longman House, Burnt Mill, Harlow
Essex CM20 2JE, England
Associated companies throughout the world

*Published in the United States of America
by Longman Inc., New York*

First published 1984

British Library Cataloguing in Publication Data
Duffus, C.M.
Carbohydrate metabolism in plants.
1. Botanical chemistry   2. Carbohydrates
—Chemical analysis   3. Plants
—Chemical analysis
I. Title   II. Duffus, J.H.
581.1'9   QK861
ISBN 0-582-44642-2

Library of Congress Cataloging in Publication Data
Duffus, C. M.
Carbohydrate metabolism in plants.

Includes bibliographical references and index.
1. Carbohydrates—Metabolism.   2. Plants—Metabolism.
I. Duffus, John H.   II. Title.
QK898.C3D83   1984   581.1'33   82-22855
ISBN 0-582-44642-2

Set in 10/12 pt Linotron 202 Times
Printed in Singapore by Selector Printing Company.

Contents

Contents   ix

Acknowledgements

We are grateful to the following for permission to reproduce copyright material:

Edward Arnold Ltd for our Fig. 8.5b from Fig. 3.7 (H. Opik 1968); J.W. Becker for our Fig. 2.13a; The Biochemical Society for our Figs. 6.6 & 6.7; C. Bucke for part of our Table 3.1 from Table 1 (Bucke & Oliver 1975 pub Springer Verlag); Chapman & Hall Ltd for our Fig. 2.11b from Fig. 4.13f (Rees 1977); D. D. Davies for our Fig. 4.5; FEBS European Journal of Biochemistry for our Figs. 2.12 from Figs. 4 (Z. Gunja–Smith *et al.*, 1970) & 5.12 from Fig. 8 (Hopp *et al.*, 1978); R. T. Giaquinta for our Fig. 3.1 from Fig. 1 (Giaquinta 1980); W. W. Norton Co Inc for our Fig. 1.4 from Fig. 4.15, p. 157 (Keeton 1980); Oxford University Press for our Figs. 8.4 & 8.5a; Pergamon Press Ltd & the authors for data in our Table 3.1 from Fig. 1, Tables 1 & 2 (Hawker & Smith 1982) & (Bird *et al.*, 1974); the Editor, *Physiologia Plantarum* (Lund University) for our Fig. 4.9 from Fig. 4, p. 729 (Tregunna *et al.*, 1966); the author, H. G. Pontis for our Table 3.2 from Table IV (Pontis & Salerno 1980); R. D. Preston for our Fig. 5.11.

Preface

This book provides an introduction to the main features of carbohydrate metabolism in higher plants.

One of the concerns of the authors is to integrate as far as possible physiological processes with biochemical events. Thus Chapter 1 begins with a brief discussion of how plant cell structure relates to function, continues with an outline of the synthesis and fate of precursor molecules produced by the chloroplast in photosynthesis and concludes with a description of some of the structural and physiological changes accompanying plant growth and development. Chapter 2 describes the structure and function of the principal plant carbohydrates and in subsequent chapters the metabolic fate of photosynthetic products is considered. For example, the synthesis and metabolism of sucrose is described in some detail, followed by a chapter concerned with the role of respiratory processes. Chapters 5 and 6 describe the mechanisms involved in polysaccharide synthesis and degradation. After considering the role of intermediates of carbohydrate metabolism in the synthesis of secondary products, the overall regulation of carbohydrate metabolism is briefly considered. Finally, in Chapter 9, the techniques available for carbohydrate analysis are assessed.

This book should be of direct interest to students taking undergraduate courses in agriculture, biochemistry, biology, botany and other biological subjects. While some elementary knowledge of botany and biochemistry is required for complete understanding, we would hope that the book will be useful to anyone interested in learning more about plant carbohydrates.

Many people have helped us at all stages of writing but we would like to thank in particular M. P. Cochrane, P. McDonald

T. ap Rees and J. R. Stark for comments and critical assessment of various parts of the manuscript. One of the authors (C. M.D.) gratefully acknowledges financial support from the Royal Society, London.

C. M. DUFFUS
School of Agriculture, University of Edinburgh

J. H. DUFFUS
Department of Brewing and Biological Sciences, Heriot-Watt University, Edinburgh

1

Overview of carbohydrate metabolism

Most plants originate from seeds which, after germination, develop into young plants or seedlings having roots, stems and leaves. This is generally followed by a period of vegetative growth during which the plant grows in size, extending its root system into the soil, and its stems and leaves upwards into the atmosphere. After some time flowers form, fertilization takes place and the seeds grow and mature.

1.1 The plant cell

1.1.1 Plant cell structure
The plant cell (Fig. 1.1) is surrounded by a cell wall which serves as protection against injury such as desiccation and osmotic shock. It also confers support and rigidity. Primary cell walls are first laid down by undifferentiated cells that are actively growing. When the cells stop growing and start to differentiate an additional cell wall may develop. This is called the secondary cell wall (Fig. 1.2). Cellulose, hemicellulose, pectins, protein and lignin are the major components of the plant cell wall. The major permeability barrier between the cell and its environment is the cell membrane or plasmalemma. Interestingly there may be connections between one cell and another called plasmodesmata which extend through the cell wall. These are lined by plasmalemma and contain threads of cytoplasm (q.v.).

Within the cell itself is a range of discrete units or organelles which themselves are separated from the cell matrix or cytosol by semi-permeable membranes. The cell contents, other than the nucleus, are generally referred to as cytoplasm. In fully developed cells as much as 80 to 90 per cent of total cell volume may be

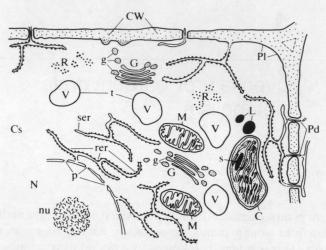

Fig. 1.1 Diagrammatic representation of the ultrastructure of a plant cell.
C, chloroplast; Cs, cytosol; CW, cell wall; G, Golgi apparatus; g, Golgi vesicle; L, lipid (oil) body; M, mitochondrion; N, nucleus; nu, nucleolus; Pd, plasmodesma; Pl, plasmalemma; p, nuclear pore; R, ribosomes; rer, rough endoplasmic reticulum; ser, smooth endoplasmic reticulum; s, starch granule; t, tonoplast; V, vacuole.

occupied by a structure called the vacuole. This is surrounded by a unit membrane called the tonoplast and functions both as a site for the storage of excretion products and as a source of water reserves.

In younger cells the most prominent cell organelle is the nucleus which contains most of the cell DNA and is concerned with cell reproduction and the overall control of cell processes. The endoplasmic reticulum is a complex network of double unit membranes within the cell. These may have small particles, called ribosomes, attached to the outer membrane. In this case the endoplasmic reticulum is known as rough surfaced. When ribosomes are absent it is referred to as smooth surfaced. It is considered that the combination of ribosomes and endoplasmic reticulum is concerned with protein synthesis and secretion across the reticulum membrane.

Of variable distribution in plant cells are the dictyosomes. These consist of several layers of membrane-bound flat vesicles or cisternae about 1–3 μm in length. One or many stacked dictyosomes constitute the Golgi apparatus of the cell. Their function

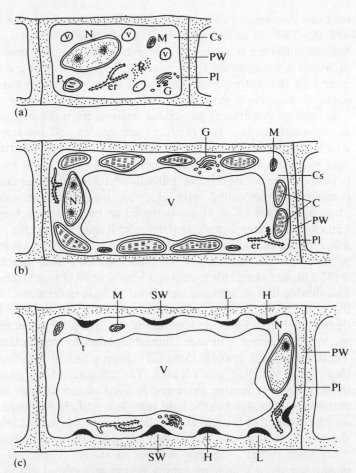

Fig. 1.2 Diagrammatic representation of some plant cell types.
(a) meristematic cell; (b) photosynthetic leaf cell (parenchyma);
(c) developing xylem cell showing secondary wall thickenings
and the beginning of lignification.
C, chloroplast; Cs, cytosol; er, endoplasmic reticulum; G, Golgi
apparatus; H, hemicellulose; L, lignin; M, mitochondrion; N,
nucleus; P, proplastid; Pl, plasmalemma; PW, primary wall; R,
ribosomes; SW, secondary wall; t, tonoplast; V, vacuole.

appears to be in secretion and also in the synthesis of polysaccharides, for example during cell wall biosynthesis.

Plant mitochondria can vary in size and shape, but on average
are cylindrical structures about $3-7 \mu$m long. Numbers are greatest
in those cells which are metabolically active. For example in maize

root cap the number of mitochondria per cell may be in the region of 1000–3000. In senescent or resting cells numbers are much less. Mitochondria are bounded by a double membrane, the inner layer of which is invaginated to form cristae. These project across the matrix of the mitochondria and appear to have small knob-like particles associated with them. The mitochondria are the site of oxidation of respiratory substrates derived from the degradation of cell constituents. The products are energy and intermediates which in turn may be used in the synthesis of new cell constituents. The enzymes of the tricarboxylic acid cycle (§1.4.1 and §4.5) are believed to be located in the mitochondrial matrix whereas those components concerned with electron transport and oxidative phosphorylation (§1.4.1) are believed to be located in the inner mitochondrial membrane. In particular it may be that the reversible ATPase thought to be responsible for ATP synthesis is present in the knob-like particles of the inner mitochondrial membrane.

The higher plant chloroplast is a lens-shaped organelle bounded by a double unit membrane and about 5–7 μm in diameter. Within the chloroplast matrix, or stroma, are flattened sac-like closed discs called thylakoids or lamellae which are piled up in circular stacks called grana. These are linked together by stroma lamellae. There might be between 15 and 20 chloroplasts in the photosynthetic cells of higher plant leaves. The enzymes of the photosynthetic carbon reduction cycle are located in the stroma, and the components involved in the light reactions and photophosphorylation are located in the thylakoids. While chloroplasts are the site of short-term storage of starch, other plastids called amyloplasts are specialized in the long-term storage of starch. These are found in storage tissues such as potato tubers and cereal grains. Like chloroplasts they are bounded by a double unit membrane, but unlike chloroplasts they do not have an internal thylakoid system. In wheat endosperm cells, where there are two types of amyloplast, A and B, the larger or A-type have a characteristic lenticular shape with a peripheral groove. A tubular complex is present inside the amyloplast membrane which may surround the granule, possibly in the groove, and may be the site of the enzymes involved in starch deposition (§5.2).

Other plant cell organelles include the microbodies which are small spherical bodies about 0.3–1.5 μm in diameter and bounded by a single unit membrane.

There are two main types of microbody. These may be distinguished by their associated enzymes and by the tissues in which they are typically found. Peroxisomes are found in photosynthesizing cells and contain a number of the enzymes involved in photorespiration (§4.7). Glyoxysomes are found in tissues active in lipid degradation, such as germinating oil seeds. They are involved in the lipid–sucrose conversion and contain those enzymes whereby fatty acids can be degraded by means of β-oxidation and the glyoxalate cycle (§3.4.2) to succinate.

1.1.2 Cell types

Plants contain a range of cell types which vary considerably in size, shape and structure. The least specialized are the meristematic cells which are small and actively dividing (Fig. 1.2a). These then grow and differentiate to produce all the other cell types. They are generally thin walled with a prominent nucleus and a few small vacuoles.

The most common cell type is the parenchymatous cell (Fig. 1.2b). These are large when mature, thin walled, relatively undifferentiated cells with a peripheral cytoplasm and large central vacuole. They may become highly specialized, for example the lamina of the leaf is mainly parenchyma (Fig. 1.4) and the cells contain many chloroplasts. Another group of cells is specialized in transport of nutrients and water within the plant. These are found in the tissues of the xylem (Fig. 1.2c) and phloem (§3.1).

1.2 The raw materials of plant growth

The growth of plants is regulated by the supply of nutrients and water as well as such factors as light intensity, day length and temperature. The nutrients required by plants include carbon dioxide and essential mineral elements.

The carbon dioxide taken in by the leaves and other green tissues is converted to sugars during photosynthesis. Mineral ions and water are taken in by the roots and transported to the growing parts including the leaves. Following the period of vegetative growth, the metabolic products, which include sucrose and amino acids, subsequently reach the developing seeds where they may be stored in the form of lipid, protein or carbohydrate and used subsequently in germination.

1.2.1 Incorporation of carbon dioxide into
photosynthetic products

Carbon dioxide is taken into the leaf cell from the atmosphere via pores in the leaf surface called stomata (Fig. 1.4). The first relatively stable product of carbon dioxide fixation in the chloroplast, catalysed by the enzyme ribulose bisphosphate carboxylase, is phosphoglyceric acid. Regeneration of the acceptor, ribulose-1,5-bisphosphate, follows within the chloroplast, catalysed by the enzymes of the photosynthetic carbon reduction cycle or Calvin cycle (Fig. 1.3). Carbon is exported from the chloroplast mainly in

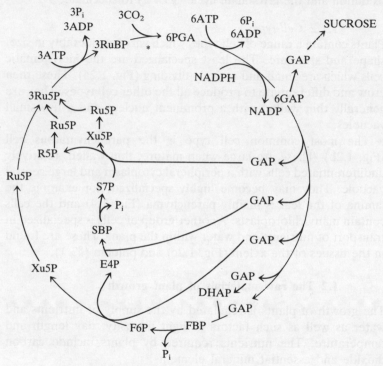

Fig. 1.3 The photosynthetic carbon reduction cycle (Calvin cycle).
(* Initial carboxylation reaction catalysed by ribulose bisphosphate carboxylase.)
DHAP – dihydroxyacetone phosphate
E4P – erythrose-4-phosphate
GAP – glyceraldehyde-3-phosphate
PGA – phosphoglyceric acid
R5P – ribose-5-phosphate
Ru5P – ribulose-5-phosphate
RuBP – ribulose-1,5-bisphosphate
SBP – sedoheptulose bisphosphate
S7P – sedoheptulose-7-phosphate
Xu5P – xylulose-5-phosphate

the form of dihydroxyacetone phosphate, much of which is converted to sucrose and utilized elsewhere. This mechanism is typical of plants such as barley, wheat and rye which are called C_3 plants, after the number of carbon atoms in the first-formed product of carbon dioxide fixation. While the Calvin cycle remains the fundamental source of reduced carbon for use in plant growth there are many variations in the overall pattern of carbon dioxide fixation. For example, in a number of tropical grasses including sugar cane (*Saccharum officinarum* L.) and maize (*Zea mays* L.) the primary carboxylation reaction is catalysed by phosphoenol pyruvate carboxylase so that the first-formed product is the C_4 acid oxaloacetate. It is for this reason that such plants are termed C_4 plants and the oxaloacetate is formed in the outer, or mesophyll cells of their leaves. The leaves of C_4 plants are distinguished from those of C_3 plants since their cells are differentiated into an inner circle of large thick-walled cylindrical cells called the bundle sheath, and an outer layer of cells called the mesophyll (Fig. 1.4). The oxaloacetate may be metabolized in a number of ways all of which involve the release of carbon dioxide and its fixation within the bundle sheath chloroplasts, as well as the regeneration of the primary carbon dioxide acceptor. For example, in maize and sugar cane, the oxaloacetate is reduced to malate within the mesophyll cell. This is then converted to pyruvate and carbon dioxide by NADP-malic enzyme in the bundle sheath cells. The pyruvate is then transported to the mesophyll where the acceptor, phosphoenolpyruvate, is regenerated by the action of pyruvate orthophosphate dikinase. The released carbon dioxide is converted to carbohydrate via the Calvin cycle in the chloroplasts of the bundle sheath cells (Fig. 1.5).

Further variation in the pattern of carbon dioxide fixation occurs in plants which are succulents and grow under conditions where water is scarce. In these, which include members of the families Cactaceae, Aizoaceae and Crassulaceae, the stomata often open only at night. While this is presumably an adaptation to prevent water loss it is associated with reduced carbon dioxide uptake during the day. In such circumstances atmospheric carbon dioxide is taken in at night and converted to C_4 dicarboxylic acids such as malic acid. Following decarboxylation, the carbon dioxide released is converted to carbohydrate during the day via the enzymes of the photosynthetic carbon reduction cycle. This type of photosynthetic metabolism is called crassulacean acid metabolism (CAM).

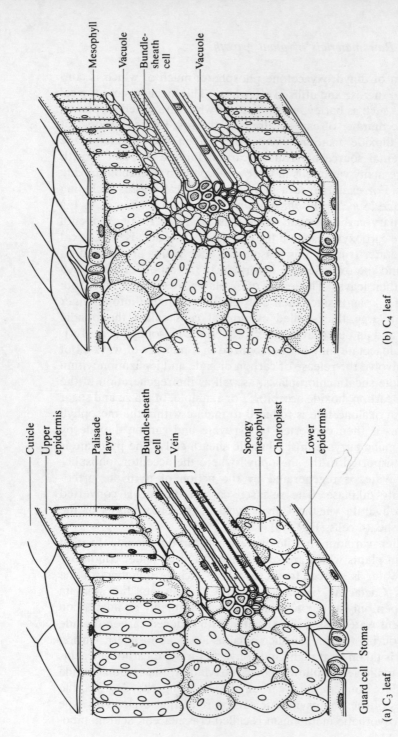

Fig. 1.4 The anatomy of C_3 and C_4 leaves. In a C_3 leaf the palisade mesophyll cells typically form a layer in the upper part of the leaf; the corresponding mesophyll cells in a C_4 leaf are usually arranged in a ring around the bundle sheath. While the bundle sheath cells of C_4 leaves have chloroplasts, those of C_3 leaves usually lack them (from Keeton, 1980).

(a) C_3 leaf

Cuticle
Upper epidermis
Palisade layer
Bundle-sheath cell
Vein
Spongy mesophyll
Chloroplast
Lower epidermis
Guard cell   Stoma

(b) C_4 leaf

Mesophyll
Vacuole
Bundle-sheath cell
Vacuole

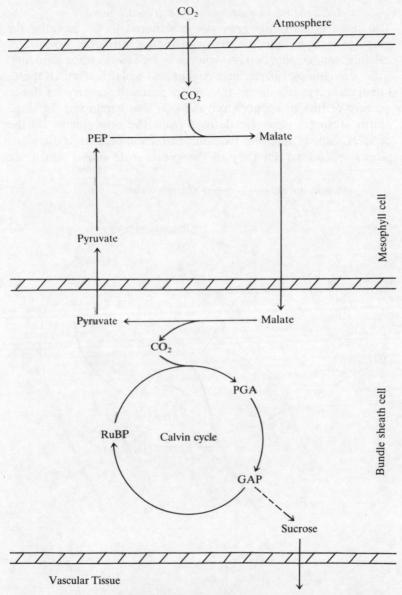

Fig. 1.5 Simplified outline of carbon dioxide fixation in leaves of
C_4 plants, e.g. maize or sugar cane.
GAP – glyceraldehyde-3-phosphate
PEP – phosphoenolpyruvate
PGA – phosphoglyceric acid
RuBP – ribulose-1,5-bisphosphate

1.2.2 *Mineral nutrition of the growing plant*

The mineral nutrients generally considered to be essential for plant growth include the major elements, nitrogen, potassium, calcium, magnesium and phosphorus as well as the trace elements, iron, manganese, boron, zinc, copper and molybdenum. Of these, nitrogen plays a dominant role in plant growth and any deficiency quickly results in reduced cell division and expansion. In some plants, nitrogen may be derived from the atmosphere by the process called nitrogen fixation. For example, in leguminous plants, bacteria (generally of the genus *Rhizobium*) which are

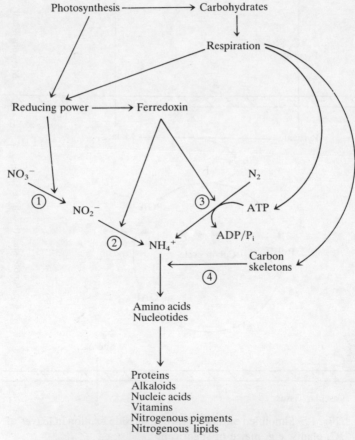

Fig. 1.6 Nitrate reduction and nitrogen fixation in relation to carbohydrate metabolism and the synthesis of plant products: (1) nitrate reductase; (2) nitrite reductase; (3) nitrogenase; (4) transaminases.

present in nodules on the roots, convert nitrogen gas to ammonia in a reaction catalysed by the nitrogenase enzyme complex. The enzymes of ammonia assimilation in the plant cell cytoplasm then convert the ammonia to amino compounds which may be transported to other parts of the plant via the xylem. Energy in the form of ATP is required for the overall process. This is presumably derived from respiratory substrates ultimately originating from reserve plant carbohydrates. Although most nitrogen is supplied as ammonia-based fertilizer, the ammonia is first oxidized to nitrate in the soil. Thus in most other plants, nitrate is the main form of nitrogen available to the root cells. Absorbed nitrate may be reduced to ammonia both in the roots and in the chloroplasts by the combined action of nitrate and nitrite reductases (Fig. 1.6). Since this conversion involves the oxidation of NADH and NADPH, a supply of respiratory substrates is again required (§1.4.1). The principal role of ammonia is as the nitrogen source for the synthesis of such molecules as amino acids, proteins and nucleic acids. The carbon required is derived from the products of carbohydrate degradation. For example, the α-keto acids, sometimes referred to as carbon skeletons, are intermediates of the tricarboxylic acid cycle (§1.4.1 and §4.5). Specifically, ammonium ions may be metabolized by either glutamate dehydrogenase or glutamine synthetase to give the amino acids glutamate and glutamine respectively (Fig. 1.7). These may then be used in the synthesis of other amino acids by means of transaminase enzymes and ultimately converted to protein.

Like nitrogen, phosphorus and sulphur are also incorporated into a number of metabolic intermediates derived fom carbohydrate oxidation. For example, the intermediates of the glycolytic pathway are all phosphorylated, the phosphate being derived from ATP. Thus there is a close relationship between the phosphate supply and carbohydrate metabolism. Phosphorus deficiency can, for example, result in an accumulation of sucrose and sometimes of starch. The requirement for sulphur is mainly in the synthesis of the sulphur-containing amino acids, cysteine and methionine, and hence its metabolism is closely related to that of nitrogen. Of the remaining essential major elements, magnesium has probably the closest relationship to carbohydrate metabolism since it is an essential cofactor for many of the enzymes involved, notably those concerned in phosphate transfer. The chief role of the essential trace elements is in biological catalysis. For example, iron has an essential role in respiration, as a constituent of the cytochromes

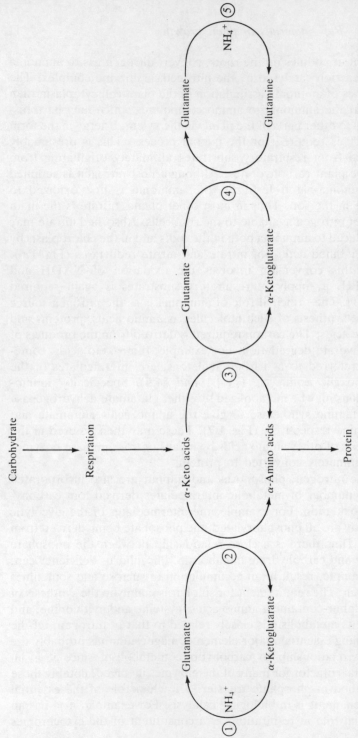

Fig. 1.7 The role of ammonium ion and carbohydrate in the synthesis of amino acids: (1) glutamate dehydrogenase; (2) (3) transaminases; (4) glutamate synthase; (5) glutamine synthetase.

and cytochrome oxidase (§1.4.1). Copper, too, is a constituent of cytochrome oxidase and, together with iron an adequate supply must be available for synthesis of this enzyme. Molybdenum deficiency in many plants may result in symptoms of chlorosis in older leaves. This is associated with high levels of nitrate in the leaves due to reduced activity of molybdenum-dependent nitrate reductase.

1.2.3 Role of water
Water is taken up by plants in relatively large amounts compared to carbon dioxide and mineral elements. Most of this, however, is lost again by evaporation from the leaves. This process is called transpiration and the consequent moistening of the leaf surface facilitates the absorption of atmospheric carbon dioxide. Water is a major component of actively growing plant cells. For example, it can account for as much as 94 per cent of the fresh weight of young, actively growing, lettuce leaves. Its functions are diverse: it is the solvent in which many substances are dissolved and in which they are transported round the plant; it provides the protons for carbon dioxide reduction in photosynthesis; it is involved directly in biochemical reactions – both as a substrate in hydrolytic reactions such as polysaccharide degradation, and as a product in condensation reactions such as polysaccharide synthesis.

1.3 The fate of photosynthetic products
While the initial products of C_3 photosynthesis are phosphorylated monosaccharides, these in turn are the precursors used by the chloroplast in the biosynthesis of a wide range of molecules, including polysaccharides, lipids and proteins. Photosynthetic products are also exported from the chloroplasts and used elsewhere for plant growth and development. Their relative contribution to the whole plant varies with its age. For example, in immature leaves much of the material remains within the leaf and is used for growth of new cells. As the leaves grow, more material is exported to the rest of the plant with younger leaves contributing relatively more to the upper parts, including the reproductive organs, and older leaves contributing relatively more to the lower stem and roots.

Only a limited number of photosynthetic products leave the chloroplast because of the selective permeability of the inner chloroplast membrane. The source of much of the carbon exported from the chloroplast, via a specific phosphate translocator, is generally considered to be dihydroxyacetone phosphate. In well-developed leaves, exporting carbon to the rest of the plant, a major function of this molecule is in the synthesis of sucrose, the form in which carbohydrate is transported in higher plants (Fig. 1.8). Dihydroxyacetone phosphate is presumably also a major substrate for respiratory metabolism from which the cell derives energy and intermediates for biosynthetic and other processes which take place outside the chloroplast.

Another product of photosynthesis which is also exported from the chloroplast is glycolic acid. This is synthesized when oxygen competes with carbon dioxide at the active site of ribulose bisphosphate carboxylase. Instead of being carboxylated, ribulose-1,5-bisphosphate is oxygenated to form phosphoglycerate and phosphoglycolate. The latter is then hydrolysed to glycolate which leaves the chloroplast and undergoes a series of reactions associ-

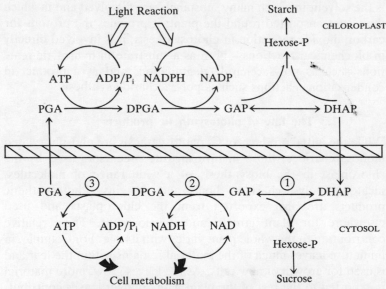

Fig. 1.8 Shuttle scheme for the export of reducing equivalents and ATP from the chloroplast during photosynthesis: (1) triose phosphate isomerase; (2) glyceraldehyde phosphate dehydrogenase; (3) phosphoglycerate kinase.

DHAP – dihydroxyacetone phosphate
GAP   – glyceraldehyde-3-phosphate
PGA   – 3-phosphoglycerate
DPGA – 1,3-diphosphoglycerate

ated with the production of carbon dioxide and the consumption of energy and reduced pyridine nucleotides. Since, in this case, the production of carbon dioxide is light-dependent, this process is termed photorespiration (§4.7).

The major fuel for the biosynthesis of most plant products is probably sucrose. For example, following degradation to α-keto acids, via the pathways of aerobic respiration it may be converted to amino acids, and hence protein, in both leaves, roots and developing seeds. Sucrose is also a precursor in the synthesis of nucleotide sugars, required for the biosynthesis of many plant polysaccharides including cellulose and starch as well as many glycoproteins, glycolipids and other glycosides. In addition, the products of sucrose metabolism may be incorporated into a wide range of plant cell components including lipids, nucleic acids and such molecules as alkaloids, vitamins, steroids and plant growth hormones (Ch. 7).

1.4 Energy production for biosynthesis

Many organisms depend solely on the oxidation of preformed materials such as carbohydrates or lipids for their energy requirements. This process, in which oxygen is consumed and the substrate oxidized to carbon dioxide and water, is generally referred to as respiration. Plants, on the other hand, although they can also obtain energy from respiratory processes, primarily derive their energy from sunlight in the light-dependent reaction called photophosphorylation.

1.4.1 Respiration

Plants can obtain energy and reducing power not only from the light reactions of photosynthesis but also from degradation of those products produced as a result of photosynthetic carbon dioxide fixation. Such degradation, or respiration, may proceed in the light but at night will presumably yield most of the energy required for maintenance of life processes. Energy from respiration must also supply much of the energy required for growth and maintenance of non-photosynthetic tissues such as those of germinating and developing seeds, roots and tubers.

The overall reaction for respiration is generally represented as the complete oxidation of a molecule of glucose:

$$C_6H_{12}O_6 + 6O_2 \longrightarrow 6CO_2 + 6H_2O + energy$$

although, as we shall see, one function of the process is to provide partially oxidized substrates to be used in many plant biosynthetic processes. Respiration itself is a sequence of enzyme-catalysed reactions which take place in a number of distinct stages (Fig. 1.9). These reactions include degradation of polymers such as polysaccharide or protein to their constituent subunits, commonly phosphorylated derivatives of glucose when starch is used as substrate. This is generally followed by further degradation via the series of reactions called glycolysis to give pyruvic acid. This molecule is then converted to acetyl coenzyme A (acetyl-CoA) which enters the tricarboxylic acid cycle (Krebs cycle) where it may be oxidized completely to carbon dioxide and water. Glycolysis and the tricarboxylic acid cycle are separated spatially, the enzymes of the former being localized in the cytosol and the latter in the mitochondria. The overall process is accompanied by the regeneration of coenzymes used up during the reaction sequence. Some of the glucose-6-phosphate formed in the first stage may be oxidized by an alternative sequence of reactions called the pentose phosphate pathway (§4.3) which essentially results in the formation of carbon dioxide and glyceraldehyde-3-phosphate. Degradation products from other sources may also feed into the overall pathway and be oxidized. For example, fatty acids may be degraded by the tricarboxylic acid cycle following oxidation to acetyl-CoA. This commonly occurs during germination of lipid-storing seeds. Proteins too may be degraded by proteases to amino acids, which in turn may be converted to intermediates of the tricarboxylic acid cycle by deamination or transamination.

The immediate products of respiration are reduced pyridine nucleotides mainly derived from the tricarboxylic acid cycle, and partially oxidized degradation products. Electrons from the reduced pyridine nucleotides are then passed down a series of electron-carrier molecules called cytochromes, and as they do so, sufficient energy is released to drive the synthesis of three ATP molecules per NADH oxidized – or two ATP molecules in the case of FADH (Fig. 1.10). The protons later combine with oxygen to produce water. The coupled reactions of electron transport and ATP synthesis are called oxidative phosphorylation and are localized in the mitochondria.

The partially oxidized products of the tricarboxylic acid cycle may be used as substrates for biosynthetic reactions. For example, acetyl-CoA is a precursor of many plant products including steroids, isoprenoids and triglycerides. Both α-ketoglutarate and

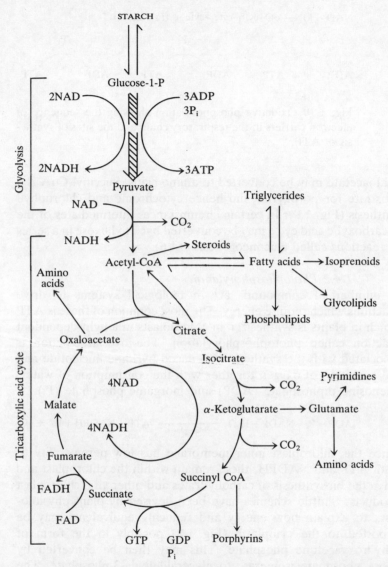

Fig. 1.9 Role of glycolysis and the tricarboxylic acid cycle in the respiratory degradation of starch. Many of the intermediates are precursors of other plant products.
GTP – guanosine triphosphate
FAD – flavin adenine dinucleotide

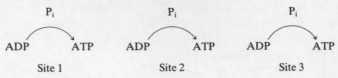

$$NAD \rightarrow FMN \rightarrow CoQ \rightarrow cytb \rightarrow cytc_1 \rightarrow cytc \rightarrow cyt(a + a_3) \rightarrow O_2$$

Site 1   Site 2   Site 3

Fig. 1.10 Oxidative phosphorylation showing the sequence of electron carriers in the respiratory chain and the sites of synthesis of ATP.

oxaloacetate may be converted to amino acids. Succinyl-CoA is a substrate for porphyrin, and hence cytochrome and chlorophyll synthesis (Fig. 1.9). In certain circumstances intermediates of the tricarboxylic acid cycle may be converted back to hexose in a series of reactions called gluconeogenesis (§4.6).

1.4.2 Photophosphorylation

A number of compounds act in biological systems to drive reactions which require energy. The most common of these is ATP which in plants is synthesized in chloroplasts in a light-dependent reaction called photophosphorylation. The overall reaction is associated with the synthesis of reduced pyridine nucleotide and the evolution of oxygen together with the consumption of water, adenosine diphosphate (ADP) and inorganic phosphate (P_i):

$$ADP + P_i + NADP + H_2O \xrightarrow[\text{chloroplasts}]{\text{light}} ATP + NADPH + H^+ + \tfrac{1}{2}O_2$$

Since the chloroplast inner membrane has low permeability to both ATP and NADPH, these remain within the chloroplast and drive the biosynthesis of carbohydrates and other vital chloroplast products. Shuttle schemes have been devised by plant physiologists to explain how energy and reducing equivalents may be exported to the cytoplasm (Fig. 1.8) possibly in the form of dihydroxyacetone phosphate. This may then be converted by triose phosphate isomerase to glyceraldehyde-3-phosphate. The next reaction is catalysed by glyceraldehyde-3-phosphate dehydrogenase with the formation of 1,3-diphosphoglycerate and one molecule of reduced pyridine nucleotide.

Effectively this represents the export of reducing power in the form of NADH. The subsequent cytoplasmic reaction yields one molecule of ATP and one of phosphoglyceric acid. The former may remain in the cytoplasm to drive energy-requiring reactions and the latter may return to the chloroplast and repeat the shuttle following internal phosphorylation and reduction to dihydroxyacetone phosphate. Of course ATP can simply be derived from dihydroxyacetone phosphate following its entry to the paths of respiration (Ch. 4).

1.5 Overall features of plant growth and development

1.5.1 The seed

The mature seed is a highly dehydrated storage organ, surrounded by a tough and generally impermeable outer layer. Differences in the structure derive mainly from variation in the relative proportions of endosperm and embryo present and also, to some extent, from variation in the thickness of the seed outer layers (Fig. 1.11a and b). All seeds have an endosperm derived from the initial nuclear fusion within the ovule (§1.5.3). The endosperm is developed probably to its greatest extent in cereal seeds where it accounts for some 70–80 per cent of final seed dry weight. Most of the starch and protein reserves of the mature seed are located in this tissue. Cereal seeds have only one cotyledon or seed leaf, and hence cereals are classified as monocotyledons. In contrast to that of cereals, the legume endosperm is short-lived and by maturity is reduced to a thin layer surrounding the embryo. Since the embryo consists largely of two cotyledons, legumes are described as dicotyledons. Legume seeds, including oil seeds such as soybean (*Glycine max*) and groundnut (*Arachis hypogaea*), as well as peas (*Pisum sativum*) and beans (*Phaseolus* spp.), differ considerably in chemical composition from cereal grains. This is a result of the

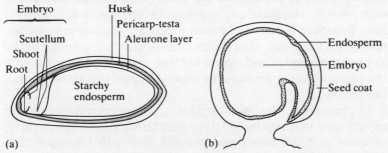

Fig. 1.11 (a) Barley (*Hordeum vulgare* L.), longitudinal section through a mature grain; (b) Pea (*Pisum sativum* L.), cross-section through a mature seed.

increased amount of embryo tissue present. Groundnut seeds, for example, may contain up to 50 per cent lipid and as much as 30 per cent protein. There are of course many different types of seed each with a characteristic chemical composition, but the cereals and legumes are of greatest economic importance since between them they provide over 50 per cent of man's dietary protein and energy.

1.5.2 Germination and growth

Germination begins with the uptake of water, and embryo growth is initally supported by reserve materials in the embryonic cells. Growth is subsequently maintained by a flow of hydrolysis products from the cotyledons or endosperm. This phase continues until the plant is established as an independent photosynthetic organism. Those regions of the plant which are actively growing, and which give rise to new cells and tissues, are called meristems (§1.1.2). These are located mainly at the tips of roots, shoots and developing branch organs. One of the early stages in cereal growth is tillering, the equivalent of branch formation. Each tiller may result in the formation of an ear. In barley, by the time six leaves are unfolded on the main stem, the potential number of grain sites has been determined. Leaves of monocotyledons, like the cereals, grow from the base, the site of the primary meristem, whereas those of the dicotyledons generally grow from the tip. Leaf growth is normally by cell expansion rather than by increase in cell number.

1.5.3 Flower and fruit formation

The initial phase of vegetative growth, characterized by stem elongation and leaf proliferation is generally followed by a reproductive phase in which flowering accompanies the termination of stem growth. The initial events following fertilization are similar in most flowering plants. The pollen tube, carrying two male nuclei, penetrates the ovary. One nucleus unites with the two polar nuclei to form the primary endosperm nucleus, and the other unites with the egg nucleus to produce the diploid zygote that develops into the embryo.

In the cereals the initial triploid endosperm nucleus divides rapidly, and in wheat by 2–3 days after fertilization there might be as many as 5,000 free nuclei present. Cell wall formation then commences and mitochondria, proplastids, endoplasmic reticulum and Golgi apparatus can be seen. Meristematic activity is in the peripheral endosperm cells which ultimately form the aleurone layer. This layer is distinguished from the starchy endosperm inside by the presence of protein-containing aleurone bodies and lipid droplets, and by the absence of starch. Embryo development commences only after at least four nuclear divisions have taken place in the endosperm. The embryo is completely surrounded by endosperm and becomes differentiated into a scutellum and a root and shoot which are separated from the nucellar epidermis and testa by a layer of modified aleurone. The mature embryo contains much lipid and protein; starch is not a major storage product. In oilseed rape, whose developmental morphology resembles that of many leguminous seeds, the endosperm is used as a nutrient supply for the growing embryo and by maturity all that remains of this tissue is a single layer of aleurone cells. Oil bodies appear in the maturing embryo of *Crambe abyssinica* quite early in development. They are smaller than other storage organelles and are surrounded by an outer membrane.

As maturation proceeds, dry weight increases steadily and reaches a maximum value. A period of dehydration accompanies the later stages of development, the seed shrinks and the outer layers harden and consolidate.

References

Bidwell, R. G. S. (1979) *Plant Physiology* (2nd edn.). Macmillan: New York.

Duffus, C. M. and Slaughter, J.C (1980) *Seeds and their Uses*. Wiley.

Hartmann, H. T., Flocker, W. J. and Kofranek, A. M. (1981) *Plant Science*. Prentice-Hall: Englewood Cliffs, New Jersey.

Keeton, W. T. (1980) *Biological Science* (3rd edn.). Norton: New York and London.

2

Carbohydrates – structure location, function

Traditionally, carbohydrates are defined as molecules containing carbon, hydrogen and oxygen in the ratio $(CH_2O)_n$ where $n \geqslant 3$. One carbon bears a carbonyl group and the others hydroxyl groups. However, many closely related compounds are often referred to as carbohydrates, although they do not quite fit this definition. Thus the term carbohydrate is often taken to include any polyhydroxy aldehyde, ketone, alcohol or acid and their simple derivatives as well as any compound that may be hydrolysed to these.

As we have seen, carbohydrate is the precursor of all plant products and with some exceptions, such as lipid-bearing seeds, it is also the major component of the plant cell.

Carbohydrates may be classified into monosaccharides, oligosaccharides, polysaccharides and an ill-defined group of compounds called complex carbohydrates.

2.1 Monosaccharides

The monosaccharides, often referred to as simple sugars, may be described as aldoses or ketoses depending on the nature of their functional group. The suffix -*ose* indicates a sugar. In turn these may be classified into trioses, tetroses, pentoses, hexoses, etc. depending on the number of carbon atoms present in the molecule. For example, aldopentoses have an aldehyde group and five carbon atoms, while ketohexoses have a ketone group and six carbon atoms.

2.1.1 Stereoisomerism
Differences between monosaccharides depend not only on variation in the number of carbon atoms present and the identity of the

active groups, but also on the presence of chiral or asymmetric carbon atoms. For example, carbon-2 (C-2) of glyceraldehyde (Fig. 2.1), probably the simplest sugar, has four different substituents. Thus two isomeric forms are possible since the groups can be arranged in two ways, each of which is a mirror image of the other. Neither, however, can be rotated so that it can be superimposed on, and hence be identical with, the other.

Such carbon atoms are said to be *chiral* or *asymmetric* and the two forms of glyceraldehyde are referred to as stereoisomers. One form is termed the D-form since it rotates plane-polarized light to the right and the other is termed the L-form since it rotates plane-polarized light to the left. By convention, the D-form is written with the hydroxyl group of C-2 at the right-hand side and the L-form with the hydroxyl group of C-2 at the left-hand side.

As the number of carbon atoms increases, so does the number of chiral carbons. In general, the number of possible stereoisomers is 2^n where n is the number of chiral carbons. Thus in the aldohexoses there are 16 possible isomers of which eight are in the L-series and eight in the D-series. Some of these are illustrated in Fig. 2.2. Some of these differ only in their configuration at a single chiral carbon. These are known as epimers. Thus D-glucose is an epimer of D-mannose and D-galactose. However, there is no such relationship between D-mannose and D-galactose.

A monosaccharide is allocated to the D- or L-series on the basis of the configuration of groups at the highest numbered chiral carbon, using glyceraldehyde as the standard. Thus in the aldohexoses, where the highest numbered chiral carbon is five, those with the same configuration at C-5 as the chiral carbon of L-glyceraldehyde are allocated to the L-series. Similarly, those with the same configuration at C-5, as the chiral carbon of D-glyceraldehyde are allocated to the D-series. Although the terms

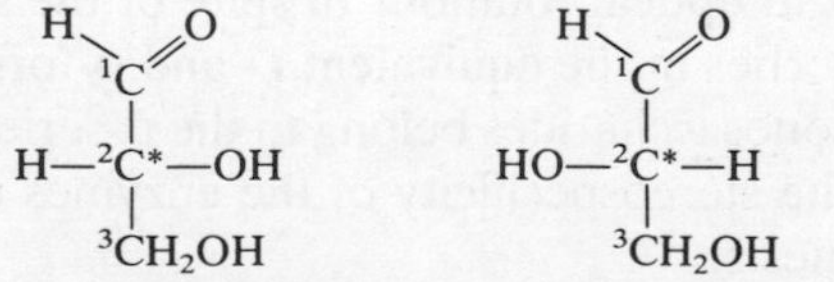

D-Glyceraldehyde   L-Glyceraldehyde

Fig. 2.1 The stereoisomers of glyceraldehyde. Carbon atoms are numbered starting from the carbonyl group (* indicates chiral carbons).

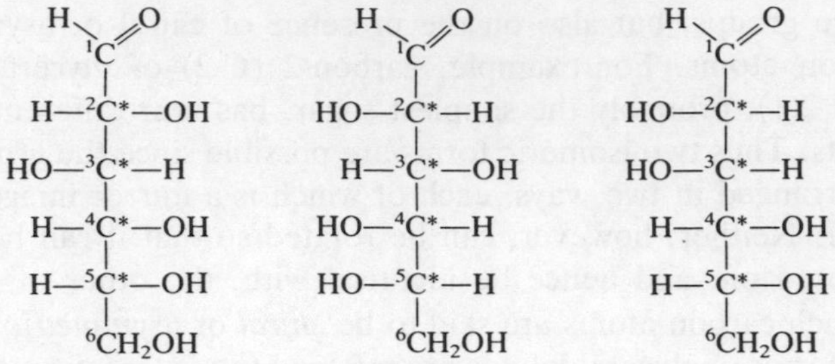

$$
\begin{array}{c}
\text{H} \diagdown \diagup \text{O} \\
{}^{1}\text{C} \\
|
\end{array}
$$

H—²C*—OH
HO—³C*—H
H—⁴C*—OH
H—⁵C*—OH
⁶CH₂OH

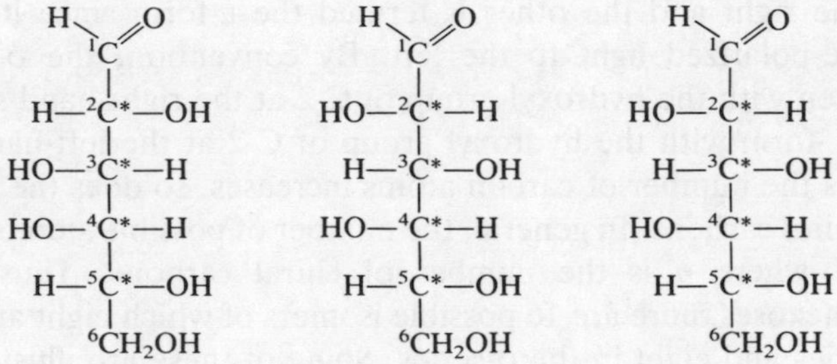

D-Glucose

HO—²C*—H
H—³C*—OH
HO—⁴C*—H
HO—⁵C*—H
⁶CH₂OH

L-Glucose

HO—²C*—H
HO—³C*—H
H—⁴C*—OH
H—⁵C*—OH
⁶CH₂OH

D-Mannose

H—²C*—OH
HO—³C*—H
HO—⁴C*—H
H—⁵C*—OH
⁶CH₂OH

D-Galactose

HO—²C*—H
H—³C*—OH
HO—⁴C*—H
H—⁵C*—OH
⁶CH₂OH

D-Gulose

HO—²C*—H
H—³C*—OH
HO—⁴C*—H
H—⁵C*—OH
⁶CH₂OH

D-Idose

Fig. 2.2 Some stereoisomers from the aldohexose series (*indicates chiral carbon). D- and L-glucose are non-superimposable mirror images. All differ only in the orientation of substituent groups about the chiral carbons.

L and D when applied to glyceraldehyde refer to the direction of rotation of plane-polarized light, this does not necessarily apply to the higher monosaccharides since the direction of rotation depends on the individual contributions from two or more chiral carbons. Thus, some may rotate light to the right and some to the left. The final direction of rotation may or may not be the same as that of highest numbered chiral carbon. In monosaccharides with more than one chiral carbon the terms L and D refer only to configuration and not to optical rotation. In spite of the similarity of structure and properties in the equivalent L- and D-forms, most naturally occurring monosaccharides belong to the D-series. This is no doubt related to the stereospecificity of the enzymes responsible for their biosynthesis.

2.1.2 Cyclic structures
The open-chain formulation in which the monosaccharides have a free carbonyl group suggests that they should behave like normal

aldehydes or ketones. However, the evidence indicates that these active groups are partially blocked. For example, they do not give Schiff's test for aldehydes. Furthermore, the aldehyde and ketone structures do not account for the change in optical rotation (mutarotation) characteristic of freshly prepared solutions of many monosaccharides.

It is now known that monosaccharides with five or more carbons usually exist as cyclic (ring) structures with an oxygen bridge between the carbonyl group and another carbon of the same molecule. Rings commonly contain either four or five carbon atoms. A five-membered ring containing four carbons and an oxygen is called a furanose ring and a six-membered ring containing five carbons and an oxygen is called a pyranose ring. Chemically, ring closure involves hemiacetal formation, where the carbonyl group (aldehyde or ketone) reacts with an alcohol:

$$R_1 - C{\overset{O}{\underset{H}{}}} + HO - R_2 \rightleftharpoons R_1 - \overset{OH}{\underset{H}{C}} - OR_2$$

  aldehyde   alcohol   hemiacetal
  *chiral carbon

This results in the formation of an additional chiral carbon, and thus two further stereoisomeric forms are possible. These are termed α- and β-forms, and when they differ at C-1 only, as in glucose, they are known as anomers. In the α-form the hydroxyl group on C-1 is *cis* to the hydroxyl on C-2, and in the β-form it is *trans*. The various forms of the monosaccharides are generally represented on paper by means of Haworth formulae. Those for glucose are shown in Fig. 2.3. In practice the thickened lines are generally omitted. The cyclic forms of some common monosaccharides are shown in Fig. 2.4.

Although ring formation removes some of the characteristic reactions of the aldehyde or ketone group, monosaccharides may show some of the properties of a carbonyl function and are often referred to as reducing sugars. Thus, they can reduce Fehling's solution and form phenylhydrazones with phenylhydrazine. This is because the α- and β-forms may be interconverted via the free aldehyde or ketone and in solution a monosaccharide may exist partly as the free aldehyde or ketone together with the α- and β-forms of the various possible rings. For example, an aqueous solution of glucose at equilibrium contains around 33 per cent

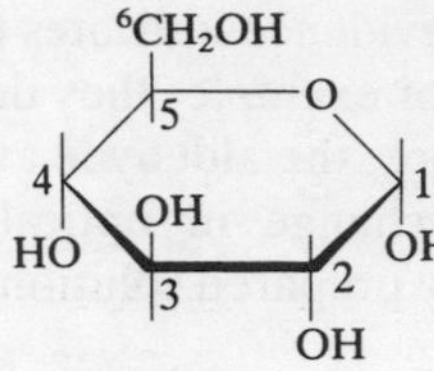

α-D-Glucopyranose

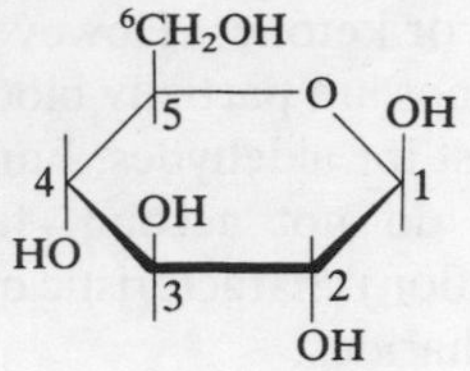

β-D-Glucopyranose

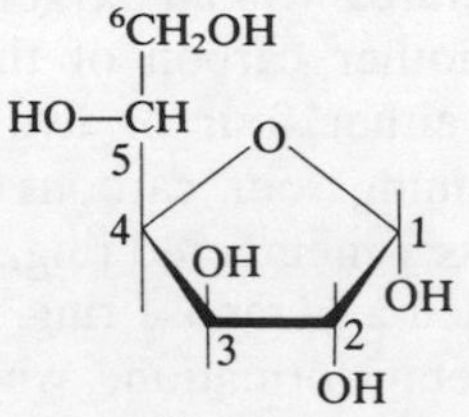

α-D-Glucofuranose

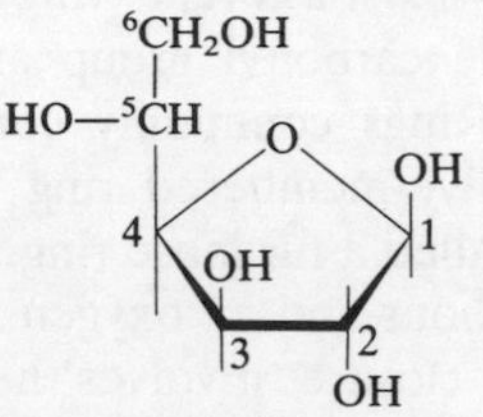

β-D-Glucofuranose

Fig. 2.3 Cyclic forms of D-glucose. In these perspective (Haworth) formulae the pyranose ring is represented as a hexagon with its lower edge nearest the observer and its upper edge furthest away. This is indicated by the slight thickening of the lower edge. The ring carbons and their substituent hydrogens are omitted for convenience. Groups attached to ring carbons are drawn either up or down depending on whether they are above or below the plane of the ring.

α-D-glucopyranose and 66 per cent β-D-glucopyranose with trace amounts of the free aldehyde and furanose forms. The absence of a conventional reaction with Schiff's reagent is due to the low concentration of free aldehyde.

The existence of mutarotation is explained by the different solubilities of the α- and β-forms. Crystalline glucose, for example, consists of α-D-glucopyranose, since this is the least soluble isomer. In aqueous solution, however, this is in equilibrium with β-D-glucopyranose. Because these are stereoisomers they have different optical rotations. That of α-D-glucopyranose is +110° and that of β-D-glucopyranose is +19°. Thus when glucose is dissolved in water the specific rotation falls until an equilibrium rotation of 53° is reached after a few hours.

2.1.3 Conformation of monosaccharides

The perspective formula (Fig. 2.3) does not give any real idea of the three-dimensional shape, or conformation, of the monosaccharides. The preferred conformations will be those in which angle

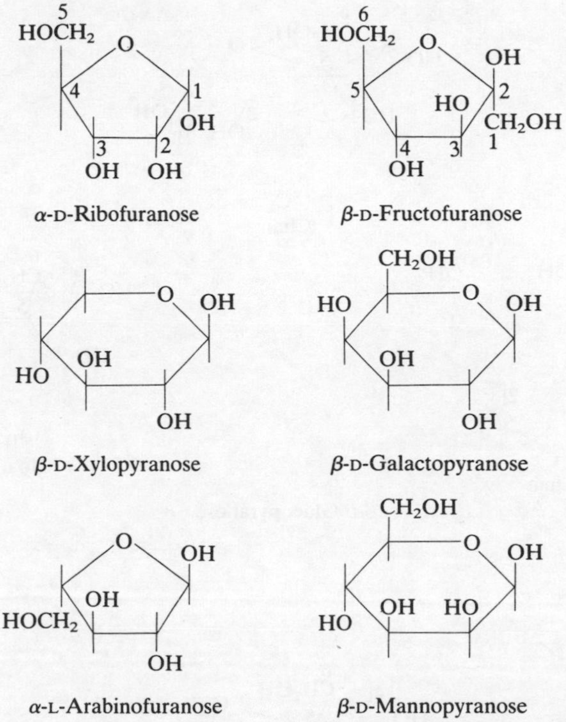

α-D-Ribofuranose

β-D-Fructofuranose

β-D-Xylopyranose

β-D-Galactopyranose

α-L-Arabinofuranose

β-D-Mannopyranose

Fig. 2.4 Cyclic forms of some common monosaccharides.

strain is least. Thus the molecule will take up that shape where the bond angles will be close to tetrahedral and the internal energy minimal. In order to achieve this, the ring cannot be flat but exists in a range of puckered or non-planar conformation. The pyranose rings, for example, can adopt eight possible forms, of which six are boat shaped and two are chair shaped (Fig. 2.5). Although six-membered rings are usually the most chemically stable, furanose rings are also widely distributed and, in the form of ribose derivatives, are a major constituent of the nucleic acids. The two major shapes of the furanose ring are *envelope* and *twist* forms of which there are 10 of each. The former has four of the ring atoms coplanar and the fifth out of plane, the latter has three ring atoms coplanar and two out of plane (Fig. 2.6).

The preferred conformation is generally one in which interaction between the substituents is minimal, that is where they project sideways (equatorial bonds) and are well separated. Those which project more or less vertically above or below the ring (axial

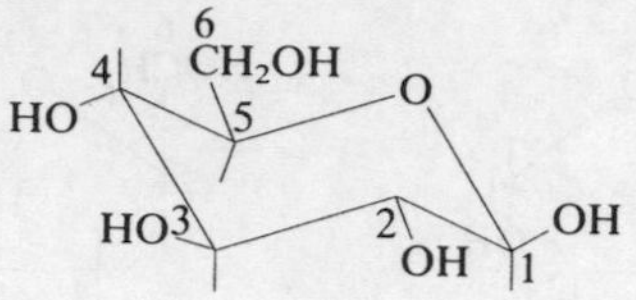

$^{4}C_1$
Chair

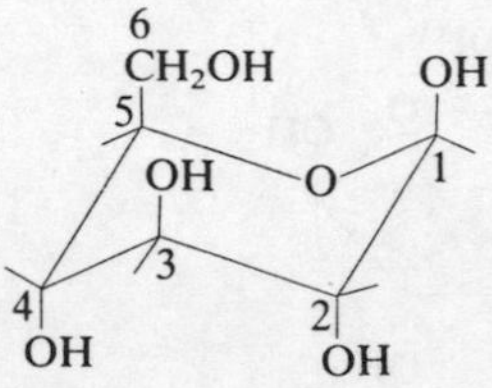

$^{1}C_4$
Chair

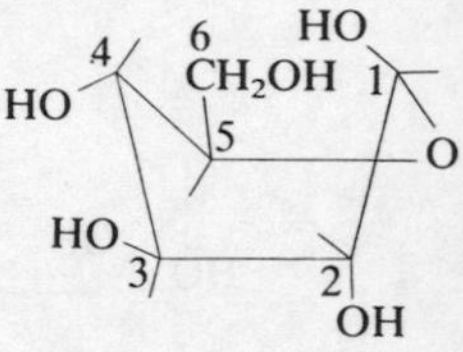

$^{1,4}B$
Boat

β-D-Glucopyranose

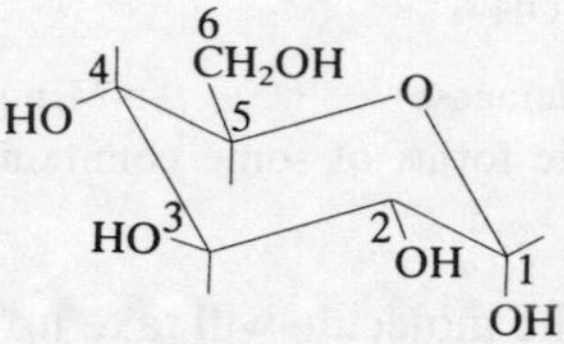

$^{4}C_1$
Chair

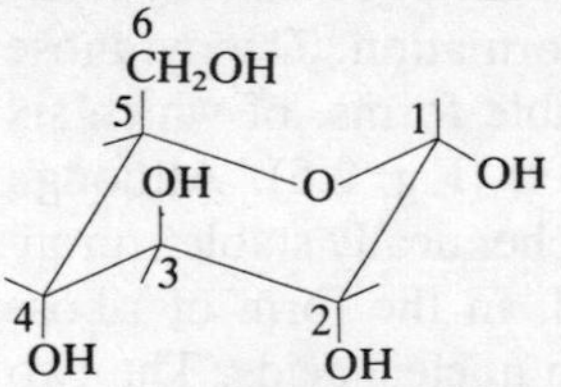

$^{1}C_4$
Chair

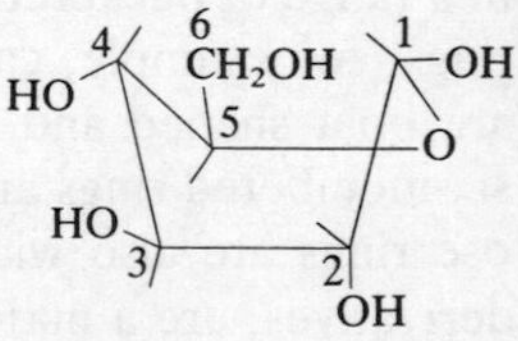

$^{1,4}B$
Boat

α-D-Glucopyranose

Fig. 2.5 Some conformations of D-glucopyranose. Some of the possible chair and boat conformations for α- and β-D-glucopyranose are shown. The preferred conformations are those free from angle strain. The ring is not flat but puckered in the shape of a chair or boat.

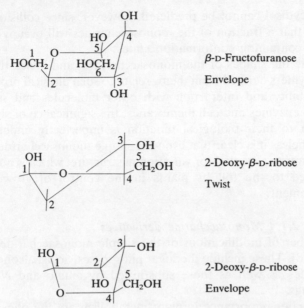

Fig. 2.6 Some conformations of furanose rings. Interconversion between the various conformational forms in the furanose series requires less distortion of bond angles, and hence less energy, than for six-membered rings. This is largely because these rings are flatter than pyranose rings. They are, therefore, more flexible, and in solution are often a mixture of several conformational forms.

bonds) are cramped and tend to repel each other (Fig. 2.7). Thus the preferred conformation of β-D-glucopyranose is the $^4C_1$ (Fig. 2.5) where all the substituents are equatorial. The hydrogen atoms are all axial but interaction between them is generally minimal because of their small size. Thus, in solution, the β-anomer is preferred since the hydroxyl of the α-anomer at C-1 is in the axial position. The precise mixture of conformations present

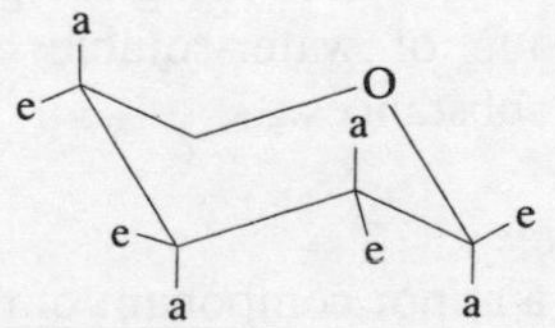

Fig. 2.7 Axial (a) and equatorial (e) bonds in the chair conformation.

in the cytosol cannot be predicted, however, since collisions will ensure that a fraction of the monosaccharides will occupy higher energy-containing conformation states.

While the shapes of the monosaccharides, and hence those of the polymers derived from them, relate to such physical properties as solubility and interaction with other molecules and surfaces such as enzymes and cell membranes, the significance of shape in relation to their biological function is imperfectly understood. Nevertheless it is clear that even the simple monosaccharides have an enormous potential for variation in structure, which is no doubt exploited to the full by plants in the control of growth and development.

2.1.4 Monosaccharide derivatives

A number of modifications of the simple monosaccharides exist (Fig. 2.8). These include the sugar phosphates, acids, alcohols and glycosides as well as those substituted by amino and *N*-acetyl groupings.

Of major importance in plant metabolism are the phosphory-lated derivatives. The first-formed stable product of photosynthe-tic carbon dioxide fixation is 3-phosphoglyceric acid (Fig. 2.8) and, as in all living tissue, phosphorylated sugars are the key intermedi-ates of carbohydrate metabolism. Those monosaccharides in which C-1 is substituted have only one anomer. This is because substitution of the anomeric hydroxyl prevents ring opening and mutarotation. At the same time substitution at the anomeric carbon means that such derivatives have no reducing properties.

There are two types of sugar acid, in one the carboxylic acid group is at C-1 and in the other the carboxylic acid group is at the highest numbered carbon atom. D-Gluconic acid is an example of the first type and, in combination with phosphate (Fig. 2.8), is an intermediate of the pentose phosphate pathway (§4.3). D-Glucuronic acid (Fig. 2.8) and D-galacturonic acid are examples of the second type, the former in combination with UDP being a precursor for pentose synthesis and the latter being the principal monosaccharide subunit of a group of water-soluble complex polysaccharides called the pectic substances.

2.1.5 The glycosidic linkage

In vivo, free monosaccharides are a minor component of the total plant cell carbohydrate. They are generally found in combination with other monosaccharides as in oligo- or polysaccharides, or in

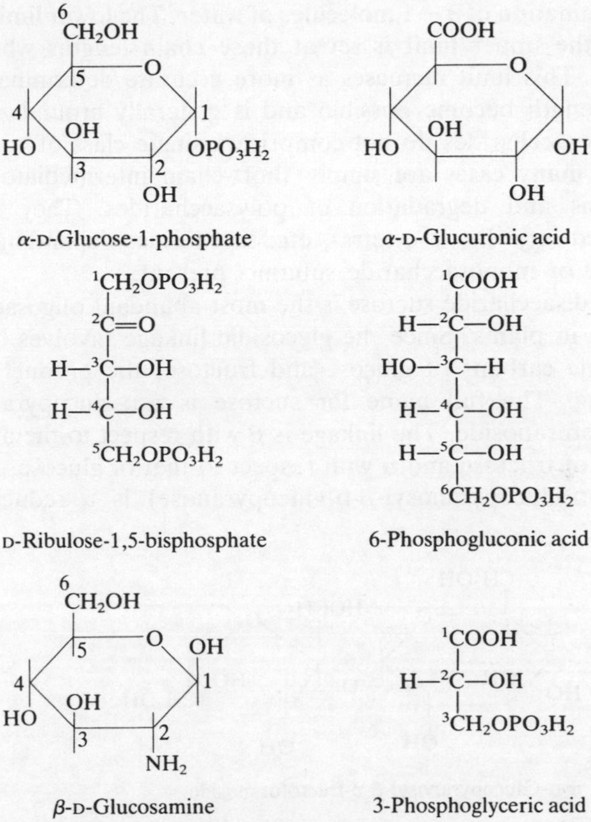

α-D-Glucose-1-phosphate

α-D-Glucuronic acid

D-Ribulose-1,5-bisphosphate

6-Phosphogluconic acid

β-D-Glucosamine

3-Phosphoglyceric acid

Fig. 2.8 Some monosaccharide derivatives.

combination with a non-carbohydrate component (aglycone) such as an alcohol or phenol. The two components are joined via the anomeric carbon through an oxygen bridge following the elimination of water. As with other C-1 substitutions, two configurations α or β are possible, depending on the original configuration of the reducing sugar. Again these are not interconverted in solution and do not show mutarotation. The bond joining the two components is referred to as a glycosidic linkage. Occasionally the two components may be linked via nitrogen or sulphur atoms (Ch. 7).

2.2 Oligosaccharides

An oligosaccharide may be defined as a small polymer formed from n monosaccharide subunits joined by glycosidic linkages with the elimination of $n - 1$ molecules of water. The lower limit for n is 2 and the upper limit is set at those chain lengths where n is known. This limit increases as more accurate determinations of chain length become possible and is generally around $n = 20$.

Oligosaccharides do not comprise a single class of compound and in many cases are simply short-chain intermediates in the synthesis and degradation of polysaccharides. They may be classified into di-, tri-, tetra-, etc. saccharides depending on the number of monosaccharide subunits present.

The disaccharide sucrose is the most abundant oligosaccharide present in plants. Since the glycosidic linkage involves both the anomeric carbons of glucose and fructose, the product is non-reducing. The full name for sucrose is α-D-glucopyranosyl-β-D-fructofuranoside. The linkage is β with respect to the anomeric carbon of fructose and α with respect to that of glucose. Maltose (4-O-α-D-glucopyranosyl-β-D-glucopyranose) is a reducing dis-

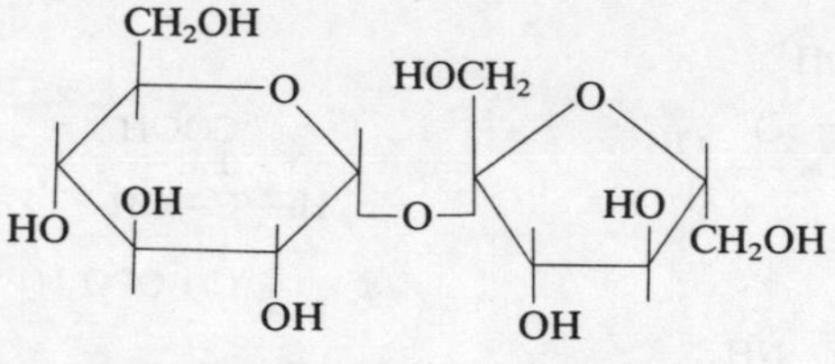

α-D-Glucopyranosyl-β-D-fructofuranoside

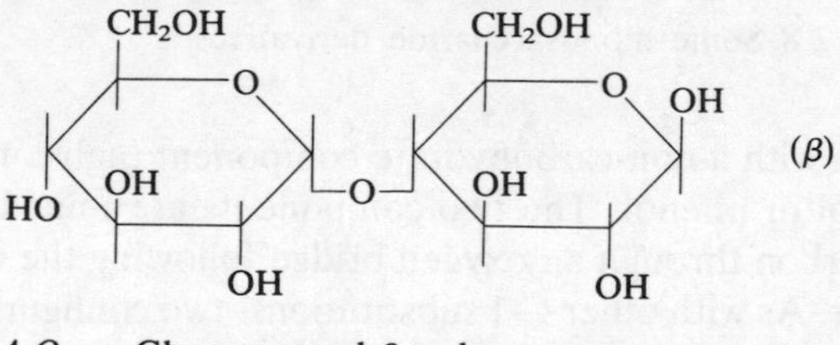

Sucrose

4-O-α-D-Glucopyranosyl-β-D-glucopyranose

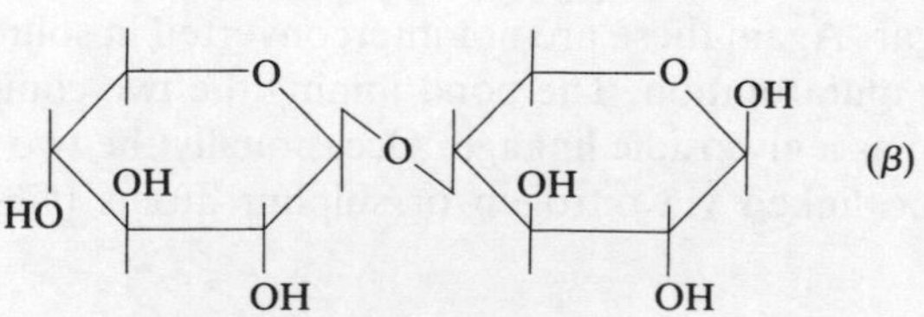

(β)   Maltose

4-O-β-D-Xylopyranosyl-β-D-xylopyranose

(β)   Xylobiose

Fig. 2.9 Some naturally occurring oligosaccharides (disaccharides).

accharide found in small amounts in many plants. In this case only the anomeric carbon of one glucose is involved (hence the term -osyl). In sucrose the term -oside at the end of the full name indicates that both anomeric carbons are involved in the glycosidic linkage.

Oligosaccharides found in higher plants include the trisaccharide raffinose and the tetrasaccharide stachyose. Structures of some disaccharides are shown in Fig. 2.9.

2.3 Polysaccharides

Polysaccharides are similar to oligosaccharides in that they are condensation polymers based on monosaccharides joined together by glycosidic linkages. They are, however, of much higher molecular weight. Many polysaccharides, including the most abundant such as starch and cellulose, contain a single type of monosaccharide subunit and are called homoglycans. Those which contain more than one type of monosaccharide subunit are called heteroglycans and include many of the plant cell wall polysaccharides. The degree of polymerization (DP), which is the number of monosaccharide subunits present, is generally of the order of 80–100. Some cellulose molecules, however, may contain as many as 5,000 residues.

2.3.1 Homoglycans

Cellulose is the most abundant naturally occurring organic compound. It is the main structural component of the plant cell wall and can be found in almost pure form in cotton fibres. It is a high molecular weight linear polymer of D-glucopyranose residues joined by β-(1→4)-glycosidic linkages (Fig. 2.10). The polymers are flat and extended ribbons in which the hydroxyl at C-3 is hydrogen bonded to the ring oxygen of the adjacent monosaccharide. Molecules in the cell wall are held together by intermolecular

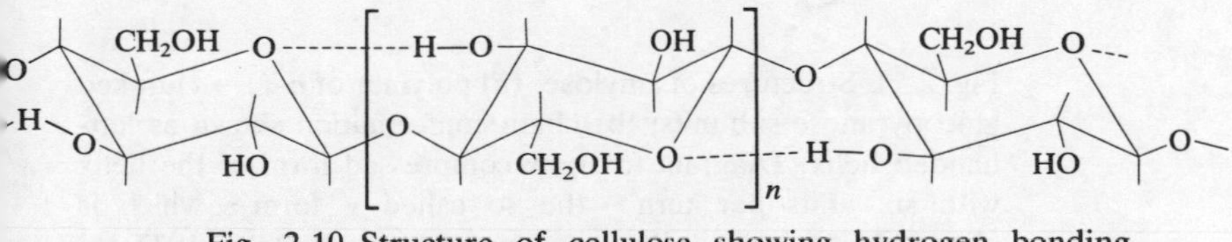

Fig. 2.10 Structure of cellulose showing hydrogen bonding between adjacent glucose residues.

hydrogen bonding and packed in parallel chains. The result is a compact, tightly bonded structure which is fibrous, insoluble, and with high strength.

Another substance with a range of interesting properties including that of selective permeability is the β-glucan, callose. This is a β-(1→3)-linked D-glucan. It is formed in response to wounding, and during the growth of pollen tubes appears to have a plugging effect. Other β-glucans form the major component of the matrix material of cereal endosperm cell walls. These are linear molecules with around 30 per cent β-(1→3)- and 70 per cent β-(1→4)-glycosidic linkages, generally randomly dispersed, and in the cell wall are firmly bound to peptide sequences.

Amylose
(a)

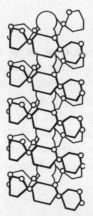

(b)

Fig. 2.11 Structures of amylose: (a) polymer of α-(1→4)-linked glucopyranose subunits; (b) chain conformation shown as left-handed helix. Diagram to show compressed form of the helix with six units per turn – the so called V form – which is obtained in certain inclusion complexes (from Rees, 1977).

Like cellulose, starch is a polymer of glucose but differs from it in the nature of the glycosidic linkage. It consists of two components, the linear polymer amylose and the branched chain polymer amylopectin, normally present in the ratio 25 per cent amylose to 75 per cent amylopectin. The former is a slightly branched but mainly linear polymer of around 1,000–2,000 D-glucopyranose units joined by α-(1→4)-glycosidic linkages (Fig. 2.11). The latter consists of chains of between 20 and 25 D-glucopyranose units in length joined together by α-(1→6)-linkages to form a branched structure (Fig. 2.12). In the plant cell the two are complexed together as discrete starch granules. Unlike cellulose, which is generally described as a structural carbohydrate, starch is readily broken down and used as an energy source for plant processes. Some attempt can be made to explain this role as a reserve material in terms of its three-dimensional structure. From studies of the complex formed between amylose and iodine it has been shown that the amylose chain is coiled into a helix with six glucose residues per turn. The hollow interior is occupied by a linear polyiodine–iodide chain and the whole structure is stabilized by hydrogen bonding between sugar residues (Fig. 2.11). It may be that when packed and folded within the starch granule such a structure is more easily accessible to hydrolytic enzymes. However, amylopectin, which is the major component of most starch granules, is unlikely to have the same degree of helical conformation since the chains are frequently interrupted by branch points (Fig. 2.12). The major structural feature of amylopectin is the very large number of non-reducing sugar residues per molecule and the short chain length. An amylopectin molecule of molecular weight 16×10^6 has about 100,000 D-glucose residues. The average chain length is between 20 and 25 residues. How the two molecules are complexed together within the starch granule is so far unknown. Phytoglycogen is a glycogen-type polysaccharide found in the endosperm of sweet corn (*Zea mays* L.) lines which are homozygous for the recessive *sugary* alleles, *su*. The average chain length is 10–14 molecules. It is thus more branched than amylopectin.

Polymers of fructose (fructans) are also found as reserve polysaccharides in the Gramineae and Compositae. Fructans may be classified into two groups according to the linkages of the principal chain. Those in the first group have β-(2→1)-linkages and include inulin and related fructans. These are found in the roots and tubers of the Compositae (Dahlia, etc. and Campanulaceae). The second group have β-(2→6)-linkages and include the

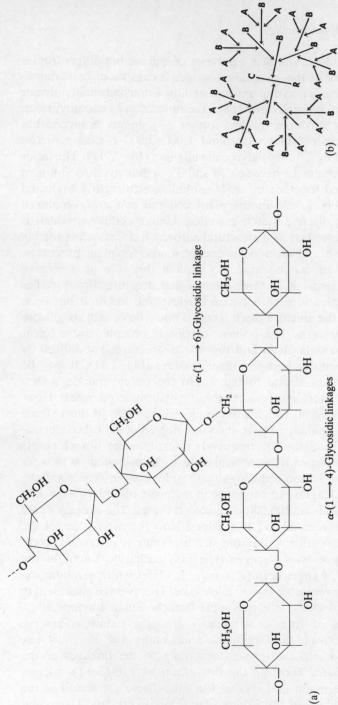

Fig. 2.12 Structure of amylopectin.

(a) Molecular structure showing α-(1→4)-glycosidic linkages and an α-(1→6)-glycosidic linkage (branch point).

(b) Revised Meyer structure showing multiple branching. A-chains are linked to the molecule by the potential reducing group. B-chains are similarly linked but additionally carry one or more A-chains. The C-chain carries the sole reducing group. R = reducing group. (From Z. Gunja-Smith, J. J. Marshall, C. Mercier, E. E. Smith and W. J. Whelan, 1970. *FEBS Letters* **12**, 101.)

In the figure:
α-(1 ⟶ 6)-Glycosidic linkage

α-(1 ⟶ 4)-Glycosidic linkages

fructans of leaves, stems and roots of the *Gramineae*. Those present in the leaves of grass crops are of particular importance during ensilage since they provide the main source of water-soluble carbohydrate for the subsequent fermentation. Strictly speaking they are not homoglycans as the terminal non-reducing monosaccharide residue is generally glucose.

2.3.2 Heteroglycans

These molecules are commonly found as constituents of cell walls, exudate gums and seed and bark mucilages. The pectic substances are water-soluble constituents of the primary cell wall. These include galacturonans, arabinans, galactans and arabinogalactans. The principal monosaccharide subunit of the rhamnogalacturonans is D-galacturonic acid and is joined by β-$(1{\rightarrow}4)$-glycosidic linkages. Rhamnose residues may be inserted in the main chain between the galacturonic acid residues. Short side chains may contain galactose, xylose and arabinose residues. They are most abundant in the peel of lemons and oranges and their gelling properties account for the success of these fruits in the making of marmalade. The carboxylate groups may be esterified with methyl groups (pectin). Any free carboxylates will be negatively charged (pectic acid) and able to bind metal ions in the cell wall such as calcium or magnesium.

Table 2.1 Some cell wall polysaccharides

Polysaccharide	Main chain monosaccharide	Side chain monosaccharide
Cellulose	D-Glucose	—
Mannans		
galactoglucomannans	D-Mannose	D-Galactose
	D-Glucose	
Pectic substances		
arabinogalactans (type I)	D-Galactose	L-Arabinose
rhamnogalacturonans	D-Galacturonic acid	D-Xylose
	L-Rhamnose	D-Galactose
		L-Arabinose
		L-Fucose
Xylans	D-Xylose	L-Arabinose
		4-Methyl-α-D-glucuronic acid
		D-Glucuronic acid
		D-Xylose

Other substances present in the cell wall of plants include the hemicelluloses which are defined essentially as a class of polysaccharide associated with cellulose and soluble in alkali. Of this group the xylans are the best characterized and are a major component of the cell walls of most flowering plants. The backbone chain consists of β-(1→4)-linked D-xylopyranose subunits. Side chains are present in varying proportions and differ in the number and type of constituent monosaccharide subunits. The hemicellulose fraction also contains galactoglucomannans and arabinogalactans (Table 2.1). Again the names refer to the principal monosaccharides of the backbone chain.

2.4 Complex carbohydrates

These may be described as carbohydrates in combination with non-carbohydrate molecules. They include the glycoproteins and glycolipids which are polymers where carbohydrate is convalently bonded to protein or lipid.

On the whole the glycoproteins are not well described in plants and the term has often been used without evidence for the presence of a covalent carbohydrate–protein link. The difficulty arises partly because the major component of the plant cell is carbohydrate, thus making characterization more difficult, and partly because a number of plant tissues contain carbohydrate-binding proteins called lectins, which may or may not be glycoproteins. Thus, for example, an electrophoretically homogeneous fraction (at pH 5.8 to 8.6) containing both carbohydrate and protein is present in *Phaseolus vulgaris* beans. However, the two components can be separated by electrophoresis at a lower pH and the free protein can be shown to have carbohydrate-binding activity.

The best known plant lectin is concanavalin A (Fig. 2.13a) which is a non-glycosylated tetrameric protein in which each subunit contains one carbohydrate binding site. In common with many lectins it can agglutinate red blood cells. This property may be related to the toxicity of many varieties of raw bean.

The primary cell walls of dicotyledonous plants contain a hydroxyproline-rich glycoprotein often referred to as extensin. Most of the hydroxyproline residues, which may account for up to 20 per cent of the total amino acid residues, are glycosylated by tri- or tetrasaccharides of arabinose. The serine residues are mostly galactosylated. The hydroxyproline regions may exist as a steep

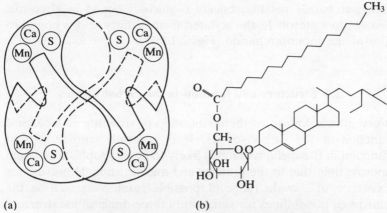

(a)   (b)

Fig. 2.13 Structures of some complex carbohydrates.
(a) Schematic representation of the concanavalin A tetramer.
Each subunit is approximately 42 × 40 × 39 Å. Ca, Mn and S
indicate the position of Ca^{2+}, Mn^{2+} and carbohydrate-specific
binding sites respectively. (From F. W. Becker, G. N. Reeke,
Jr, B. A. Cunningham and G. M. Edelman, 1976. *Nature* **259**,
406.)
(b) Acylated sitosteryl glucoside.

left-handed helix giving a rigid molecule with a rod-like shape. It
may be that this glycoprotein forms part of a cross-linked matrix
with cellulose and hemicellulose in the cell wall. Other extracellular hydroxyproline-containing glycoproteins include soluble arabinogalactan proteins (AGPs or β-lectins). The main chain of the
polysaccharide component has a DP of around 50 β-(1→3)-linked
D-galactose residues with galactosyl side chains attached at C-6.
L-Arabinose residues may be attached to terminal galactose residues as well as to the side chain residues. The hydroxyproline-
rich protein component is thought to contain around 100 amino
acids and is attached to the galactan chain by glycopeptide linkage
between hydroxyproline and galactose.

Galactolipids are the major glycolipids of plants and are found
usually as the mono- and digalactosyl glycerol derivatives. They
are found as a major component of the plasmalemma (cell
membrane) and chloroplast membrane lipids. It is likely that the
galactosyl residues are located on the outer aqueous phase and the
lipid moiety in the inner hydrophobic region of the membranes.
Other plant glycolipids are the steryl glycosides. These consist of a

monosaccharide residue, usually D-glucose, bound in glycosidic linkage to a sterol. In the acylated form, a fatty acid is bound to C-6 of the monosaccharide (Fig. 2.13b).

2.5 Structure and function in the carbohydrates

Very little is known of the relationship of structure to biological function in the carbohydrates. It is generally considered that function in the carbohydrates is likely to be less sophisticated and specific than that in the proteins and nucleic acids. However, the existence of a wide range of possible isomers as well as the enormous possibilities for variation in three-dimensional structure suggests that the biological diversity of the carbohydrates has not always been appreciated.

In animals, carbohydrate is transported as glucose in the blood stream. In most plants, however, the main transport carbohydrate is sucrose. The advantage to the plant of using sucrose may be a function of its non-reducing properties. Thus it is less reactive and less easily metabolized than glucose. Plants are much more vulnerable than animals to damage from external forces, such as predators and disease. The use of a relatively inactive molecule such as sucrose means that it is less likely to be metabolized during damage, either by the plant's own enzymes or by those of the predators or infective agents. A major function of glucose in animals is as a rapidly and easily available source of energy for use in an emergency. This is not an important requirement in plants and any advantage is presumably outweighed by the protective effect of the (1→2) glycosidic linkage.

Other examples exist where function may be related to structure. The long chains of β-(1→4)-linked glucopyranose subunits in cellulose give rise to a ribbon-like and easily packed conformation where the hydroxy groups are available for both inter- and intramolecular bonding. Thus the structure is strong and resistant to degradation. On the other hand, the properties of starch, which is also a homoglycan of D-glucopyranose residues may be explained in part by the helical nature of the amylose component (§2.3.1)

Similarly, studies of orientated pectic acid fibres indicate how their three-dimensional structure relates to their gel-forming properties. From X-ray diffraction patterns and computer model building it can be shown that polygalacturonic acid chains adopt a buckled or zigzag shape held together by crystalline polygalacturonate junctions where several chains align. The occasional presence of a rhamnose residue prevents gel aggregation by causing 'kinking' of the chain, or by introducing branch points.

References

Aspinall, G. O. (1970) *Polysaccharides*. Pergamon.

Aspinall, G.O. (ed.) 1982 *The Polysaccharides*, Vol. 1. Academic Press.

Aspinall, G. O. (1981) Constitution of plant cell wall polysaccharides, in *Encyclopedia of Plant Physiology* (*Plant Carbohydrates II*), Vol 13B (W. Tanner and F. A. Loewus, eds.). Springer-Verlag: Berlin.

Candy, D. J. (1980) *Biological Functions of Carbohydrates*. Blackie.

Preiss, J. (ed.) (1980) Carbohydrates: structure and function, in *The Biochemistry of Plants*, Vol. 3 (P. K. Stumpf and E. E. Conn, eds.). Academic Press: New York.

Preston, R. D. (1979) Polysaccharide conformation and cell wall function, *Ann. Review of Plant Physiology* **30**, 55–78.

Rees, D. A. (1977) *Polysaccharide Shapes*. (Outline Studies in Biology). Chapman & Hall.

3

Sucrose metabolism

In most plants sucrose is the form in which carbohydrate is transported from the sites of synthesis to the sites of utilization or storage. It is the most common disaccharide of plant tissues and is the precursor of most of the carbon-containing molecules found in plants. For example, it is the primary precursor of the lipid, protein, and carbohydrate stores of mature seeds; it moves out from these stores during germination to provide energy and substrates for cell growth and differentiation in the absence of photosynthesis; and it is presumably the immediate source of energy for maintenance of plant life during periods of darkness.

3.1 Sucrose translocation

As the plant grows, material is exported from the leaves to the places of storage and growth. Those tissues where new organic materials are synthesized or where storage materials are mobilized are termed sources. These include the leaves as well as germinating seeds. The sites where the transported material is utilized are termed sinks and include meristems and cotyledons or endosperms of developing seeds. Material is transferred to sinks from sources by the process of translocation. In vascular plants this consists of two main pathways. The first is via the cytoplasm of the plant cell (symplast) and includes long-distance transport through the cells of the phloem as well as transfer over short distances via intercellular connections called plasmodesmata (Fig. 1.1). The main conducting unit of the phloem is the sieve element which includes specialized cells called sieve cells and sieve-tube elements. The sieve elements are elongated and arranged end-to-end in longitudinal rows to make sieve tubes. Associated with these are companion cells which may be concerned in the secretion of enzymes into the sieve elements. The direction of flux within the phloem is mainly from sources to sinks. The second pathway is located in the extracellular tissues (apoplast) of the plant and serves to conduct water, ions and some organic substances from the roots to the upper transpiring parts of the plant. These specialized tissues are called the xylem and consist of thick-walled conducting cells (Fig. 1.2c). These include vessels, which are large cells with no

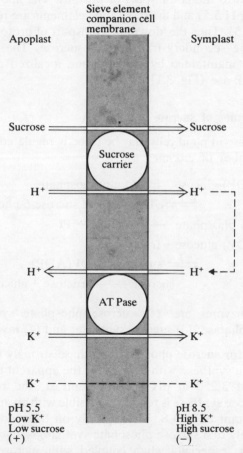

Fig. 3.1 Model of sucrose loading across the sieve element–companion cell plasmalemma. Potassium entry into the phloem may occur via a H^+/K^+ exchanger or by equilibration in response to the inside negative membrane potential (from Giaquinta, 1980).

end walls that form tubes running up the length of the stem, and tracheids, which are smaller cells with end walls. Carbohydrate is present only in trace amounts in xylem. The greater part of carbohydrate translocation thus takes place in the phloem. The loading of material into the sieve element–companion cell complex thus generates the increased osmotic pressure to drive the mass flow of assimilates. Phloem loading is a selective process requiring metabolic energy and although the mechanism of sucrose uptake into the sieve elements is not yet clear, it is likely that it may be coupled to the cotransport of protons. The apoplast is relatively acidic (pH 5.5) and the sieve-tube elements are relatively alkaline (pH 8.5). Thus the 'downhill' transport of protons may be coupled to the secondary transport of sucrose. The proton gradient may be maintained by a membrane localized proton-translocating ATP-ase (Fig. 3.1).

3.2 Enzymes of sucrose metabolism

The level of sucrose in plant cells may be directly regulated by the activity of a number of enzymes:

$$UDP(ADP)\text{-glucose} + \text{fructose-6-phosphate} \underset{1}{\rightleftharpoons} UDP(ADP) + \text{sucrose-6-phosphate}$$

$$\text{sucrose-6-phosphate} \xrightarrow{\;2\;} \text{sucrose} + Pi$$

$$UDP(ADP)\text{-glucose} + \text{fructose} \underset{3}{\rightleftharpoons} \text{sucrose} + UDP(ADP)$$

$$\text{sucrose} \xrightarrow{\;4\;} \text{fructose} + \text{glucose}$$

These enzymes are: (1) sucrose phosphate synthase; (2) sucrose phosphatase; (3) sucrose synthase; and (4) invertase.

The equilibrium for sucrose phosphate synthase strongly favours sucrose phosphate synthesis with a value for the apparent equilibrium constant of 3,250 at pH 7.5. In contrast, the reaction catalysed by sucrose synthase is readily reversible with an apparent equilibrium constant of 1 to 8. Thus, purely on thermodynamic grounds, it is likely that sucrose phosphate synthase is involved in sucrose synthesis, especially when coupled with sucrose phosphatase, which is an essentially irreversible reaction in the direction of sucrose synthesis. There is some evidence to suggest that sucrose synthase activity is greater in tissues concerned in sucrose utilization, such as developing cereal endosperms and low in ex-

Table 3.1 Activities of sucrose-metabolizing enzymes in various tissues

| Tissue | Enzyme activity (μmol h^{-1} g^{-1} fr. wt.) | | | |
	Sucrose synthase	Sucrose phosphate synthase	Sucrose phosphatase	Ref.
Developing bean cotyledons	15.6	9	132	1
Developing maize endosperm	40	2.4	44	1
Spinach leaves (England)	0.4	25.0	n.d.	2
Spinach leaves (Australia)	n.d.	3.0	29	3
Pennisetum purpureum leaves	0.7–13.8	77–161	n.d.	4
Germinated maize endosperm	3.5	1.6	16.8	1
Germinating castor bean endosperm	18.6	16.9	165	1

(1) J. S. Hawker, 1971. *Phytochem.* **10**, 2313; (2) I. F. Bird, M. J. Cornelius, A. J. Keys and C. P. Whittingham, 1974. *Phytochem.* **13**, 59; (3) J. S. Hawker and Smith, 1982. Unpublished; (4) C. Bucke and I. R. Oliver, 1975. *Planta.* **122**, 45.

tracts of photosynthesizing tissues thus indicating that this enzyme may be involved in sucrose cleavage. However, in many plant tissues all three enzyme activities can be detected regardless of whether the tissue is concerned in storage or degradation of carbohydrate (Table 3.1). It is, therefore, difficult to conclude whether sucrose synthase is engaged in sucrose cleavage or sucrose synthesis, or even whether the sucrose phosphate synthase/ phosphate system is solely concerned in sucrose synthesis.

Sucrose may be hydrolysed to glucose and fructose by invertase. Both acid and neutral invertases are present in plant tissues and in general appear to be associated with sucrose uptake. For example, sucrose derived from leaf photosynthesis can be stored in sugar cane stems only after first being hydrolysed by an acid invertase localized in the cell walls (§3.8) Invertase may be involved in the formation of reducing sugars in potato tubers as a result of sucrose hydrolysis during cold storage (§3.5).

3.3 Sucrose synthesis in leaves

Sucrose is derived from dihydroxyacetone phosphate exported from the chloroplast during photosynthesis (Fig. 3.2). In the

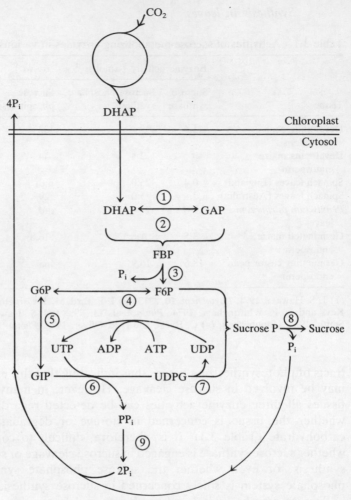

Fig. 3.2 Possible pathway for sucrose synthesis in leaves.
DHAP – dihydroxyacetone phosphate
GAP   – glyceraldehyde-3-phosphate
FBP   – fructosebisphosphate
F6P   – fructose-6-phosphate
G6P   – glucose-6-phosphate
G1P   – glucose-1-phosphate
UDPG – uridinediphosphate-glucose
PP_i – pyrophosphate
(1) triosephosphate isomerase; (2) aldolase; (3) fructose-
bisphosphatase; (4) phosphohexoisomerase;   (5) phospho-
glucomutase; (6) UDP-glucose pyrophosphorylase; (7) sucrose
phosphate synthase: (8) sucrose phosphatase; (9) pyrophos-
phatase.

presence of cytoplasmic triose phosphate isomerase the dihydroxy-acetone phosphate equilibrates with glyceraldehyde-3-phosphate. These combine via an aldol condensation to form fructose-1,6-bisphosphate. This may then be converted successively to fructose-6-phosphate, glucose-6-phosphate and glucose-1-phosphate in reactions catalysed by fructosebisphosphatase, phosphohex-isomerase and phosphoglucomutase respectively. Glucose-1-phosphate then combines with UTP in a reaction catalysed by UDP-glucose pyrophosphorylase to give UDP-glucose and pyrophosphate. A glucose residue is then transferred from UDP-glucose to fructose-6-phosphate with the formation of sucrose phosphate. This reaction is catalysed by sucrose phosphate synth-ase. Finally, free sucrose is released by the action of sucrose phosphatase. In the presence of pyrophosphatase, two phosphates are released from the pyrophosphate and four phosphates are then available for return to the chloroplast where they may be utilized in the regeneration of triose phosphate following photophosphory-lation.

3.3.1 Regulation of sucrose synthesis

Clearly the rate of sucrose synthesis is dependent on the supply of triose phosphate and hence on the rate of photosynthesis. At the same time the rate of sucrose utilization in the sink may affect the supply of primary substrates. However, the chloroplast membrane is impermeable to sucrose – hence its use as an osmoticum in chloroplast isolation – and, therefore, presumably it cannot have a direct effect on triose phosphate synthesis. Any effect must, therefore, be on cytoplasmic reactions. There is some evidence for regulation at the level of either sucrose phosphate synthase or sucrose phosphatase. Sucrose is an inhibitor of sucrose phosphate synthase (see Table 3.2) and sucrose phosphatase. Any increase in cytoplasmic sucrose levels, due to reduced uptake or sink activity might therefore result in increased triosephosphate concentration as a result of a mass action effect. Of course a simple mass action effect might well operate in the absence of any enzyme effects. High cytosolic levels of triose phosphate will inhibit net export of this molecule from the chloroplast and hence may favour starch synthesis. At the same time, any accumulation of the intermedi-ates of sucrose metabolism will result in reduced levels of cytosolic inorganic phosphate. Since photosynthesis consumes inorganic phosphate, lowered phosphate levels may reduce photosynthesis,

Table 3.2 Effect of oligosaccharides on the activity of wheat germ sucrose phosphate synthase (Pontis and Salerno, 1980)

Oligosaccharide (50 mM)	UDP formed (nmol)	Activity (%)
—	19.5	100
Sucrose	10	52
Raffinose	20	102
Maltose	20	102
Cellobiose	19.5	100
Trehalose	19.6	100
Melibiose	20	102

possibly by a reduced ATP/ADP ratio or by a direct effect on ribulosebisphosphate carboxylase activity (see Herold, 1980).

On the other hand, when sucrose is rapidly removed to the sites of sink activity and metabolized to other products, the inhibition of sucrose phosphate synthase and sucrose phosphatase will be removed, and recycling of the released inorganic phosphate to the chloroplast will ensure a continued supply of ATP for triose phosphate synthesis. Thus sink activity might regulate the rate of photosynthesis itself.

3.4 Sucrose synthesis in germinating seeds

During germination in cereal grains the products of starch digestion in the endosperm are transported to the growing embryo via the shield-shaped scutellum. The role of the scutellum is to absorb these products and convert them to sucrose. Subsequently the sucrose may be transported to the embryo via the phloem which connects the two tissues. The products of carbohydrate degradation are probably glucose, maltose and some oligosaccharides (Ch. 6). Glucose may be absorbed by the scutellum both passively and by active transport. Maltose is probably hydrolysed to glucose by α-glucosidase soon after uptake. Early after the start of germination in maize, activities of sucrose phosphate synthase/phosphatase and sucrose synthase can be detected although the reaction in rice scutellum seems to favour the former enzymes and in this tissue fructose-6-phosphate rather than fructose is the preferred donor.

In a similar way the lipid reserves of oil-bearing seeds such as sunflower, castor bean or groundnut are broken down during germination to sucrose via a complex series of reactions involving the co-operation of four discrete cell compartments, the oil bodies, the glyoxysomes, the mitochondria and the cytosol (Fig. 3.3). The first event is the degradation of lipid by lipases to give fatty acids and glycerol in the oil bodies. This is followed by fatty acid oxidation and synthesis of succinate via the glyoxylate cycle, which takes place in the glyoxysomes. These are distinctive organelles surrounded by a single unit membrane, with an amorphous matrix, and about 1 μm in diameter. Oxaloacetate derived from succinate oxidation in the mitochondria then enters the cytosol where it is converted to sucrose via the reactions of gluconeogenesis (§4.6). The glycerol derived from the initial lipolysis may be phosphorylated to α-glycerophosphate (glycerol-3-phosphate) in the cytosol, then converted to dihydroxyacetone phosphate in the mitochondria and finally may enter the pathways of sucrose synthesis following conversion to fructosebisphosphate.

3.4.1 Lipid degradation

Most of our information relating to the conversion of lipid reserves to carbohydrate is derived from the work of Beevers and his colleagues using germinating castor beans. It is likely, however, that the overall pattern is similar in most germinating seeds.

Within two days of imbibition (water uptake) in castor beans, lipase activity can be detected in the endosperm. Mobilization of the reserve lipid commences on about the third day and by seven days the endosperm is completely liquefied and the products have been taken up by the growing cotyledons. Triglycerides are the major reserve lipids in seeds and the products of lipase activity are successively diglycerides, monoglycerides and finally glycerol, together with three free fatty acids:

$$
\begin{array}{cccc}
\text{O} & \text{O} & \text{O} & \\
\| & \| & \| & \\
CH_2OC\!-\!R_1 & CH_2OC\!-\!R_1 & CH_2OC\!-\!R_1 & CH_2OH \\
| \quad \text{O} & | \quad \text{O} & | & | \\
| \quad \| & | \quad \| & | & | \\
CHOC\!-\!R_2 \longrightarrow & CHOC\!-\!R_2 \longrightarrow & CHOH \longrightarrow & CHOH \\
| \quad \text{O} & | & | & | \\
| \quad \| & | & | & | \\
CH_2OC\!-\!R_3 & CH_2OH & CH_2OH & CH_2OH
\end{array}
$$

triglyceride   diglyceride   monoglyceride   glycerol

+ R_3COOH + R_2COOH + R_1COOH
fatty acid   fatty acid   fatty acid

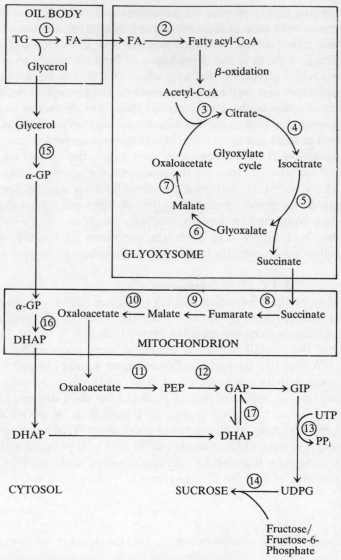

Fig. 3.3 Sucrose synthesis in the endosperm of germinating castor beans.

DHAP – dihydroxyacetone phosphate
FA   – fatty acid
GAP   – glyceraldehyde-3-phosphate
α-GP   – glycerol-3-phosphate
G1P   – glucose-1-phosphate
PEP   – phosphoenolpyruvate

The released fatty acids, which may include both saturated and unsaturated fatty acids, are then degraded by a series of reactions called β-oxidation in which two carbon units are sequentially removed in the form of acetyl-CoA. Before oxidation, unsaturated fatty acids require rearrangement to a form suitable for β-oxidation. For example, the polyunsaturated fatty acid, linoleic acid, a major component of the triglycerides of cereal grains, oilseeds and legumes, is converted from a *cis,cis*-1,4-pentadiene system to a *cis,trans*-butadiene system by the enzyme, lipoxygenase before β-oxidation:

$$CH_3(CH_2)_4-CH=CH-CH_2-CH=CH-(CH_2)_7COOH$$

cis   *cis*

O_2 LIPOXYGENASE

$$CH_3(CH_2)_4-CH=CH-CH_2-CH=CH-(CH_2)_7COOH$$

cis   *trans*

Initially it was assumed, by analogy with the mammalian system, that the reactions of β-oxidation were localized in the mitochondria. However, it was later found that these reactions were also present in the glyoxysomes. The fatty acids, following esterification with CoA, are postulated to enter the glyoxysomes and undergo conversion to acetyl-CoA via the reactions of the glyoxylate cycle.

3.4.2 The glyoxylate cycle

The glyoxylate cycle is a modified form of the tricarboxylic acid cycle in which the steps involving carbon dioxide release are

---

Caption to Fig. 3.3 (*cont.*)
PP_i – pyrophosphate
UDPG – uridinediphosphate glucose
(1) lipases; (2) thiokinases; (3) citrate synthase; (4) aconitase; (5) isocitrate lyase; (6) malate synthase; (7) malate dehydrogenase; (8) succinate dehydrogenase; (9) fumarase; (10) malate dehydrogenase; (11) PEP carboxykinase; (12) reversal of glycolysis; (13) UDP-glucose pyrophosphorylase; (14) sucrose synthase (or sucrose phosphate synthase and sucrose phosphatase); (15) glycerol kinase; (16) glycerol-3-phosphate dehydrogenase; (17) triosephosphate isomerase.

bypassed. Thus for every two acetyl-CoA molecules entering this cyclic series of reactions, one C_4 dicarboxylic acid can be released as a substrate for sucrose synthesis (Fig. 3.3).

The enzymes catalysing the entry of acetyl-CoA into the glyoxylate cycle are citrate synthase and malate synthase. Citrate synthase catalyses the condensation of acetyl-CoA with the acceptor oxaloacetate. One molecule of citrate is thus formed. The equilibrium is well in favour of citrate synthesis. Following conversion of citrate tô isocitrate in a reaction catalysed by aconitase, succinate and glyoxylate are formed in a freely reversible reaction catalysed by isocitrate lyase.

At this stage succinate leaves the cycle and glyoxylate condenses with a second molecule of acetyl-CoA to form malate. This reaction, driven by the hydrolysis of the thioester, is highly exergonic and effectively irreversible. The acceptor oxaloacetate is then regenerated from malate by the action of malate dehydrogenase. *In vitro* at pH 7.0 the equilibrium is in favour of malate formation, however, during periods of rapid lipid degradation and ample supply of substrate, oxaloacetate is rapidly removed thus allowing the oxidation to continue. Both malate synthase and isocitrate lyase are considered to be characteristic of the glyoxylate cycle and are used as marker enzymes for the glyoxysome. It is clear, from experiments in which labelled acetate was fed to slices of endosperm from germinating castor bean, that acetate is utilized exclusively in the glyoxylate cycle and none in the tricarboxylic acid cycle. In other tissues, however, such as maize scutellum and marrow seedlings, some acetate may be metabolized further by the tricarboxylic acid cycle and eventually enter the pathways of amino acid and protein synthesis.

3.4.3 The fate of succinate

The conversion of succinate to sucrose takes place via a complex sequence of enzyme-catalysed reactions of which a major part involves the reversal of glycolysis. The first step in the sequence is catalysed by succinate dehydrogenase, an enzyme not present in the glyoxysome but localized on the mitochondrial membrane. Thus it is postulated that the succinate formed as a result of the isocitrate lyase reaction leaves the glyoxysome and enters the mitochondria for further metabolism. This may be oxidized to oxaloacetate by a partial sequence of the tricarboxylic acid cycle and, following release to the cytosol, may then be converted to phosphoenolpyruvate in a reaction catalysed by phosphoenolpyruvate carboxykinase. Subsequent reactions involve the conversion of phosphoenolpyruvate to glucose-1-phosphate by the reversal of glycolysis (§4.6). Sucrose is then derived from glucose-1-phosphate via UDP-glucose as described above for leaves (§3.3). Again, the relative contributions of sucrose phosphate synthase and sucrose synthase are unknown. Germinating castor bean endosperms have comparatively high activities of these enzymes as well as sucrose phosphatase (Table 3.1).

More than 70 per cent of the carbon derived from stored triglyceride during germination in castor beans may be converted to sucrose. This is then taken up by the cotyledons and transported to the sink (radicles) and utilized in seedling growth.

3.5 Sucrose synthesis during sweetening of potato tubers

The reducing sugar content of potatoes is of key importance if they are to be processed into fried products.. In the manufacture of potato crisps a limit of 2.5–3 mg reducing sugars per gram fresh weight is set, since above this level the potatoes darken unacceptably due to a Maillard reaction taking place between the aldehyde groups of the reducing sugars and the amino groups of the amino acids. This appears to be due to the production of glucose and fructose from sucrose in a reaction catalysed by invertase. The effect is promoted by storage at low temperatures when both sucrose and reducing sugars accumulate. Thus, while it is desirable to store potatoes at low temperatures to reduce losses due to respiration, sprouting and disease, higher temperatures are advisable if the potatoes are to be used for crisping. As the temperature is raised, invertase activity decreases, possibly as a result of inhibition by an endogenous proteinaceous inhibitor, and respiration rates increase. Thus glucose and fructose levels are decreased due to reduced production coupled with increased rates of degradation through respiratory pathways. Sucrose levels also decrease. It seems, therefore, that at low temperatures, e.g. 2 °C, sucrose synthesis is favoured, probably at the expense of stored starch. As the temperature rises, sucrose is utilized, apparently in the direction of starch synthesis.

It has been suggested by ap Rees and colleagues that cold-induced sucrose synthesis may be attributed, at least in part, to differential sensitivity of glycolysis to low temperature. Both phosphofructokinase and pyruvate kinase are more sensitive to cold than are the other enzymes involved in hexosephosphate metabolism. It was also shown that in mature potato tubers phosphofructokinase exerts a dominant role in regulating entry into glycolysis and that pyruvate kinase, by determining levels of glycolytic intermediates, may influence phosphofructokinase activity indirectly. Thus, reduction in activity of both enzymes at low temperature could lead to a decrease in hexose phosphate degradation. It may be then that the accumulated hexose phosphates are used in sucrose synthesis. At higher temperatures the inhibition will be relieved, hexose phosphates are consumed in respiration and sucrose levels fall.

3.6 Sucrose utilization in developing seeds

In developing cereal grains it can only be assumed that sucrose is the main carbon source for the synthesis of storage material since it has not so far proved possible to analyse the phloem contents and identify the molecules entering the grain. Furthermore, it is still not clear whether sucrose enters the developing grains unchanged. In wheat, for example, when sucrose was supplied as ^{14}C-fructosyl sucrose, there was little randomization of ^{14}C between the fructose and glucose moieties of sucrose extracted from the pericarp and endosperm. Hence sucrose may enter the wheat grain from the phloem without hydrolysis. In maize, on the other hand, sucrose is hydrolysed by invertase to glucose and fructose during entry to the growing endosperm.

Oddly enough, although the factors regulating the conversion of sucrose to storage materials in developing seeds are of enormous commercial interest, the metabolic interconversions involved are not fully understood. Much of the sucrose entering the developing cereal grain is converted to starch which is the major component of yield in this crop. It seems to be generally agreed that most of the incoming sucrose (with the exception of the early stages of maize endosperm development) is converted to UDP-glucose and fructose by UDP-dependent sucrose synthase:

$$\text{sucrose} + \text{UDP} \rightleftharpoons \text{UDP-glucose} + \text{fructose}$$

Although the affinity of the enzyme is greatest towards UDP-glucose, other nucleosidediphosphate glucoses may be synthesized such as ADP-glucose, CDP-glucose and GDP-glucose. Some of these may be utilized in the biosynthesis of cell wall polysaccharides (§5.4). Thus the products of sucrose metabolism in developing grains include sugar nucleotides, fructose and some glucose. If

UDP-glucose is indeed the major product then, since the greater part of starch synthesis is catalysed by ADP-glucose-dependent starch synthase (§5.2.3) it seems likely that much of the UDP-glucose formed is converted first to glucose-1-phosphate and then to starch via ADP-glucose and ADP-glucose pyrophosphorylase as shown in Fig. 5.6. Presumably some UDP-glucose is converted directly to starch via UDP-glucose-dependent starch synthase. Fructose, formed as a product of both sucrose synthase and invertase activity, may be metabolized to glucose-1-phosphate via the action of fructokinase, glucose-6-phosphate ketoisomerase and phosphoglucomutase. It too may then enter the pathways of starch synthesis. At the same time, energy is required to drive the biosynthetic reactions associated with the deposition of storage material. Thus some of the glucose-1-phosphate no doubt enters the pathways of respiratory metabolism (Fig. 3.4; Fig. 5.6).

The role of sucrose in the synthesis of protein and lipid during seed development is less well understood. The protein synthesized in developing seeds contains the full range of amino acids whereas the amino acids entering the developing seed from the phloem are limited largely to aspartate/asparagine and glutamate/glutamine. Thus, much synthesis and rearrangement of amino acids must occur within the developing seeds themselves. Presumably most of the required carbon skeletons are derived from intermediates of carbohydrate degradation since levels of sucrose in the phloem most likely greatly exceed those of the amino acids. The fatty acids of storage triglycerides (§3.4.1) are most likely derived from acetyl-CoA which in turn is a product of pyruvate oxidation. Sucrose is assumed to be the major source of pyruvate following conversion to fructose-6-phosphate. The pyruvate is then degraded via the glycolytic pathway. The α-glycerophosphate, with which the fatty acids are ultimately esterified, is derived from dihydroxyacetone phosphate in a reaction catalysed by glycerol-3-phosphate dehydrogenase. Some of the reactions that may be involved in the conversion of sucrose to protein and lipid are shown in Fig. 3.4.

3.6.1 Regulation of sucrose utilization
The capacity of the plant to supply sucrose to developing cereal grains, and possibly in other species, appears in most circumstances to exceed the ability of the grain to use it. It is, therefore, suspected that factors operating in the grains themselves limit the deposition of storage material. These might include the rate of

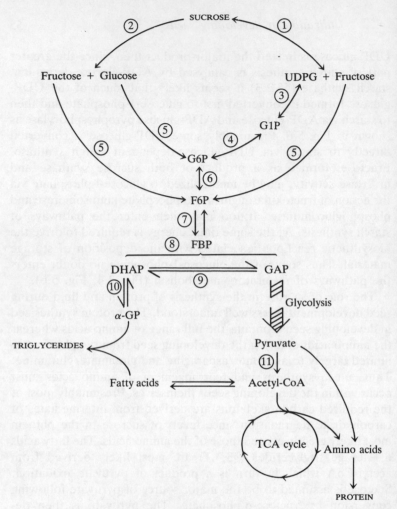

Fig. 3.4 Hypothetical scheme for the conversion of sucrose to protein and lipid during cereal grain development.

DHAP – dihydroxyacetone phosphate
FBP – fructosebisphosphate
F6P – fructose-6-phosphate
α-GP – glycerol-3-phosphate
G1P – glucose-1-phosphate
G6P – glucose-6-phosphate
GAP – glyceraldehyde-3-phosphate
UDPG – uridinediphosphate glucose
(1) UDP-dependent sucrose synthase; (2) invertase; (3) UDP-glucose pyrophosphorylase; (4) phosphoglucomutase; (5) hexo-kinase; (6) phosphohexoisomerase; (7) phosphofructokinase; (8) aldolase; (9) triosephosphate isomerase; (10) glycerol-3-phosphate dehydrogenase; (11) pyruvate dehydrogenase.

sucrose transport into the cells of the growing endosperm or cotyledons, the rate of enzyme-catalysed reactions involved in sucrose utilization, the extent of grain respiratory processes and even perhaps the elastic properties of the seed outer layers. Little is known of the regulation of sucrose uptake into the developing cells. Once inside the cells, however, it is assumed that, at least in the stage of most rapid growth, sucrose is quickly metabolized to starch, lipid or protein. Clearly a key metabolite of sucrose utilization is glucose-1-phosphate, derived either from sugar nucleotides or fructose. Since the transglycosylation reaction from sucrose to ADP is strongly inhibited by UDP, the formation of ADP-glucose must depend very closely on intracellular levels of UDP. What evidence there is suggests that in cereal grains UDP levels exceed those of ADP. Furthermore, the major pyrophosphorylase activity of higher plants is UDP-glucose-dependent as is sucrose synthase and so it is assumed that any regulation of sucrose utilization occurs at the level of UDP-dependent sucrose synthase and UDP-glucose-dependent pyrophosphorylase.

The plant UDP-glucose pyrophosphorylases are highly specific towards UDP-glucose, UTP and glucose-1-phosphate. Significantly they are strongly inhibited by UDP-glucose and it may be that this acts as an allosteric regulator *in vivo*. Thus UDP-glucose may regulate its own synthesis, as for example when levels increase due to a reduction in glucose-1-phosphate utilization or an increase in the supply of sucrose.

3.7 Sucrose utilization in leaves

In the early stages of growth, leaves are net importers of the products of photosynthesis. As development proceeds, however, their photosynthetic capacity increases and they become net exporters of photosynthetic products. In sugar beet leaves this change in function from source to sink occurs when the leaf is 40 to 50 per cent expanded (see Giaquinta, 1980). In the younger or sink leaves, sucrose arrival is followed by hydrolysis and the appearance of hexoses, after 1 to 2 h. Some of the hexoses are phosphorylated and either enter the glycolytic pathway or are used in biosynthetic reactions. Within 5 h more than half the carbon entering the leaf is incorporated into starch and protein. As the leaf matures, sucrose levels rise and the leaf becomes a net exporter. Interestingly, this is apparently not due to any decrease in invertase levels, which remain substantially unchanged. Sucrose synthase activity too remains unchanged. Significantly, however, sucrose phosphate synthase is not detectable in sink leaves but is present in source leaves. It may be, therefore, that the transition from sink to source is related to increased levels of sucrose synthesis catalysed by sucrose phosphate synthase.

3.8 Sucrose storage

The events associated with the unloading of sucrose from the sieve tubes and its subsequent metabolism in the sink region are probably best understood in developing sugar cane stalks. After hydrolysis in the apoplast by invertase, tightly bound to the cell wall, glucose and fructose are transported into the cytosol of the storage cells where they may be rapidly reconverted to sucrose by a sequence of reactions involving hexokinase, phosphohex-oisomerase, phosphoglucomutase, UDP-glucose pyrophosphory-lase, sucrose phosphate synthase and sucrose phosphatase. The final reaction is accompanied by transfer of the sucrose into the vacuole.

On the other hand the mechanism of sucrose unloading and storage in sugar beet roots appears to be rather different. In this case it appears that sucrose enters the vacuole without hydrolysis. The high vacuolar concentrations suggest that transport across the tonoplast involves active transport, possibly similar to that already described for phloem loading (§3.1), and coupled to the cotrans-port of protons. Similarly, in germinating castor bean seedlings, sucrose is absorbed by the cotyledons and transported to the radicles without hydrolysis. Sucrose levels within the vacuole are thought to be controlled by a cytoplasmic neutral invertase (pH 7.0) in the case of mature sugar cane stalks, and by sucrose synthase in the case of sugar beet.

References

Beevers, H. (1980) The role of the glyoxylate cycle, in *The Biochemistry of Plants*, Vol. 4 (P. K. Stumpf and E. E. Conn, eds.). Academic Press: New York.

Dixon, W. L. and ap Rees, T. (1980) Carbohydrate metabolism during cold-induced sweetening of potato tubers, *Phytochemistry* **19**, 1653–6.

Duffus, C. M. and Cochrane, M. P. (1982) Carbohydrate metabolism during cereal grain development, in *The Physiology and Biochemistry of Seed Development, Dormancy and Germination* (A. A. Khan, ed.). Elsevier/North Holland Biomedical Press: The Netherlands.

Giaquinta, R. T. (1980) Translocation of sucrose and oligosaccharides, in *The Biochemistry of Plants*, Vol. 3 (P. K. Stumpf and E. E. Conn, eds.). Academic Press: New York.

Herold, A. (1980) Regulation of photosynthesis by sink activity – the missing link, *New Phytologist* **86**, 131–44.

Nishimura, M. and Beevers, H. (1979) Subcellular distribution of gluconeogenetic enzymes in germinating castor bean endosperm, *Plant Physiol.* **64**, 31–7.

Pontis, H. G. and Salerno, G. L. (1980) Regulation of sucrose levels in plant cells, in *Mechanisms of Saccharide Polymerization and Depolymerization* (J. J. Marshall, ed.). Academic Press: New York.

Whittingham, C. P., Keys, A. J. and Bird, I. F. (1979) The enzymology of sucrose synthesis in leaves, in *Encyclopedia of Plant Physiology*, Vol. 6, Photosynthesis II (M. Gibbs and E. Latzko, eds.). Springer-Verlag: Berlin.

4

Respiratory metabolism

The energy and intermediates used in plant biosynthetic reactions are derived either directly from photosynthesis or from the respiration of carbohydrate, protein and lipid. Carbohydrate is the major contributor to plant respiratory activity and the role of protein and lipid, except in certain specialized tissues, is a minor one. The contribution of respiration, often referred to as 'dark' respiration in order to distinguish it from photorespiration, to overall plant growth and metabolism has been subject to much speculation and experiment, but is still poorly understood. One problem is to assess the extent of respiration in the light. In this context respiration may be defined as the degradation of metabolites via glycolysis and/or the oxidative pentose phosphate pathway, the products being oxidized by the tricarboxylic acid cycle and the resultant pyridine nucleotides used in the synthesis of ATP via oxidative phosphorylation in mitochondria.

It is likely that requirements for energy and reducing power in the light are fully met by photosynthesis. However, particularly in young growing photosynthetic tissues, where high rates of biosynthesis occur, respiratory activity is presumably necessary for the supply of carbon skeletons for biosynthetic reactions. In older tissues, however, there may be a reduced requirement for such precursors. The difficulty in determining experimentally the extent of 'dark' respiration in the light stems from the fact that in green tissues at least, photosynthesis, photorespiration and 'dark' respiration may be operating simultaneously. Thus, the oxygen uptake of 'dark' respiration must be distinguished from the light-dependent oxygen uptake of photorespiration in a cell which is rapidly evolving oxygen in photosynthesis. Similarly, the carbon dioxide evolution of 'dark' respiration must be distinguished from the light-dependent carbon dioxide evolution of photorespiration against a background of carbon dioxide fixation in photosynthesis.

Most studies suggest that 'dark' respiration continues in the light but that rates may be less than those operating in the dark. Because of the experimental difficulties, much of the work on higher plant respiration has been carried out using non-photosynthetic tissues.

4.1 Origin of respiratory substrates

The primary substrates of carbohydrate respiration are hexose phosphates, which originate from the degradation of sucrose and reserve polysaccharides such as starch and fructan. They may also be formed from intermediates of the tricarboxylic acid cycle via gluconeogenesis (§4.6) or from dihydroxyacetone phosphate exported from the chloroplast during photosynthesis. Subsequent degradation of hexose phosphate then takes place via glycolysis and/or the oxidative pentose phosphate pathway.

Although protein and amino acids can be respired in higher plants, their contribution to overall respiration is thought to be a minor one. The respiratory substrates in this case would be intermediates of the tricarboxylic acid cycle derived from amino acids following transamination and deamination (Fig. 4.1). These intermediates may then be completely or partially oxidized to carbon dioxide or used as precursors in other biosynthetic reactions. In developing fruit and seeds, for example, it is likely that nitrogen is not supplied in the form of a complete range of amino acids in the correct proportions but rather as a few amino acids which require much metabolic transformation, probably via the tricarboxylic acid cycle, before incorporation into new protein. However, in this tissue, as in others such as senescing leaves and germinating seeds where protein degradation takes place, the relative importance of amino acid respiration as opposed to the use of amino acids in biosynthetic reactions is not known. In excised starved leaves, for example, as much as 40 per cent of the respired carbon dioxide may be derived from protein. Whether this is the case *in vivo* remains to be established.

The contribution of lipids to plant respiration is also difficult to assess. The major storage lipid of higher plants is triglyceride which, following β-oxidation would be converted to acetyl-CoA. Since the enzymes of β-oxidation are located in the microbodies or glyoxysomes and those of the tricarboxylic acid cycle are located in

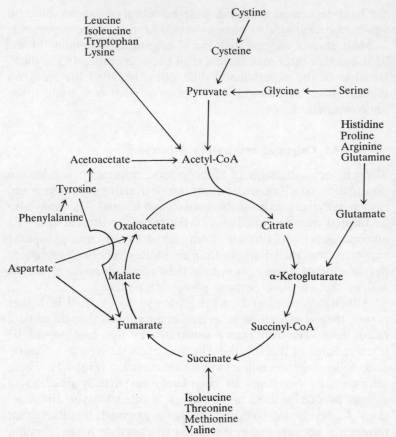

Fig. 4.1 Degradation of amino acids to respiratory intermediates.

the mitochondria, it seems unlikely that acetyl-CoA derived from lipid breakdown ever enters the tricarboxylic acid cycle directly. Oxidation of acetyl-CoA in the tricarboxylic acid cycle probably only takes place after it has been through the glyoxylate cycle.

In seeds such as castor bean where stored triglyceride is converted to sucrose during germination (§3.4) it seems that very little is oxidized in respiration. With marrow cotyledons, although some of the products of lipid breakdown may be metabolized in the tricarboxylic acid cycle, the intermediates produced are not completely respired but most likely used in biosynthetic reactions. Little information is available concerning lipid breakdown in tissues other than fat-storing seeds and present evidence suggests that lipid does not in general make a significant contribution to overall plant respiratory processes.

Thus it seems that under most conditions carbohydrate is the major source of energy and reducing power for plant metabolic activity.

4.2 The glycolytic pathway

Conventionally the glycolytic pathway (Fig. 4.2) is described as a series of enzyme-catalysed reactions in which hexose phosphate is degraded to pyruvate. All the available evidence suggests that it is universal in higher plants and that the overall sequence of reactions is broadly similar to that found in other living systems.

In general the greater part of carbohydrate oxidation in plant cells is catalysed by glycolysis but with a small but significant contribution from the pentose phosphate pathway (Fig. 4.5).

Evidence for the existence of the pathway in plants includes the identification of the enzymes involved, together with their substrates. Further support comes from experiments in which the expected intermediates were formed following feeding of labelled substrates. The reversible interconversion of hexose phosphates is catalysed by phosphohexoisomerase and the fructose-6-phosphate formed is then converted to fructose-1,6-bisphosphate in the presence of ATP and phosphofructokinase:

$$^{2-}O_3POCH_2 \quad \overset{O}{\diagup} \quad CH_2OH$$
$$HO \diagup OH$$
$$OH$$

fructose-6-phosphate

$$\xrightarrow[\text{phosphofructokinase}]{\text{ATP} \quad \text{ADP} \atop \searrow Mg^{2+} \nearrow}$$

$$^{2-}O_3POCH_2 \quad \overset{O}{\diagup} \quad CH_2OPO_3^{2-}$$
$$HO \diagup OH$$
$$OH$$

fructose-1,6-bisphosphate

This reaction is essentially irreversible under physiological conditions and is highly sensitive to changes in cellular concentration of a number of key metabolites. For example plant phosphofructokinases may be inhibited by citrate, ATP, ADP and phosphoenolpyruvate and stimulated by magnesium and monovalent cations.

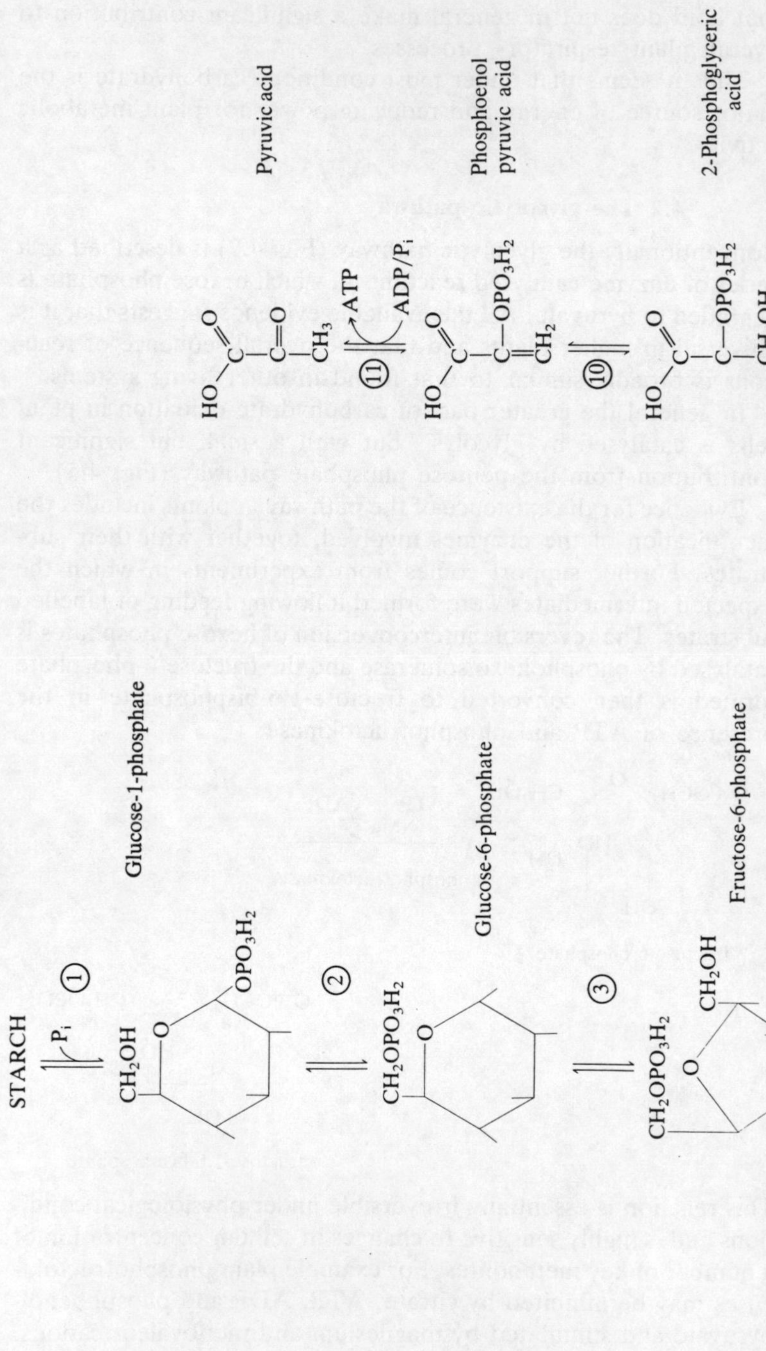

STARCH

① P_i

Glucose-1-phosphate

CH₂OH

OPO₃H₂

②

Glucose-6-phosphate

CH₂OPO₃H₂

③

Fructose-6-phosphate

CH₂OPO₃H₂

CH₂OH

Pyruvic acid

Phosphoenol pyruvic acid

2-Phosphoglyceric acid

⑪

ATP

ADP/P_i

⑩

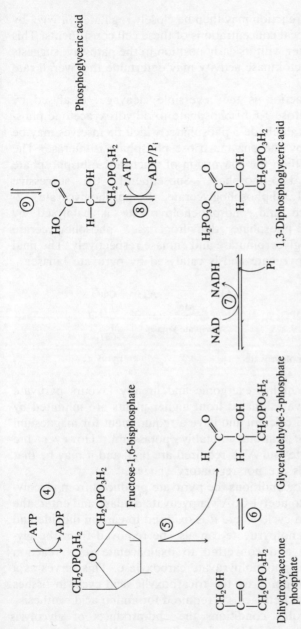

Fig. 4.2 The glycolytic pathway. (1) phosphorylase; (2) phosphohexoisomerase; (3) phosphohexoisomerase; (4) phosphofructokinase; (5) aldolase; (6) triosephosphate isomerase; (7) glyceraldehyde-3-phosphate dehydrogenase; (8) phosphoglycerate kinase; (9) phosphoglyceromutase; (10) enolase; (11) pyruvate kinase.

The rate of this reaction may then be closely regulated *in vivo* by changes in the local concentrations of these cell constituents. This evidence, together with its early position in the pathway, suggests that phosphofructokinase activity may determine the overall rate of glycolysis.

The next reaction is the reversible cleavage, catalysed by aldolase, of fructose-1,6-bisphosphate to dihydroxyacetone phosphate and glyceraldehyde-3-phosphate, which themselves may be interconverted by the enzyme triose phosphate isomerase. The overall effect is then the conversion of fructose-1-6-bisphosphate to glyceraldehyde-3-phosphate. Subsequently the successive formation of 1,3-diphosphoglycerate, 3-phosphoglycerate, 2-phosphoglycerate and phosphoenolpyruvate is catalysed by glyceraldehyde-3-phosphate dehydrogenase, phosphoglycerate kinase, phosphoglyceromutase and enolase respectively. The final reaction yields pyruvate and is catalysed by pyruvate kinase:

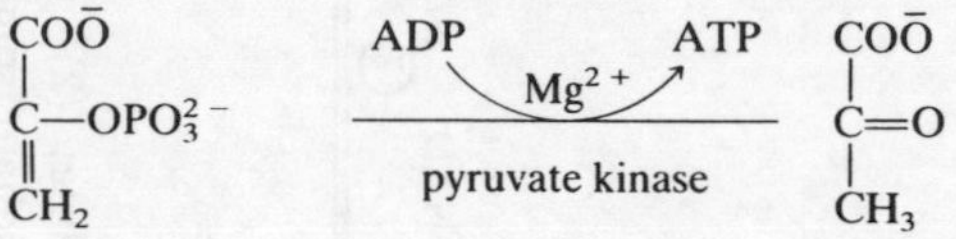

$$
\begin{array}{c}
\text{CO}\bar{\text{O}} \\
| \\
\text{C}-\text{OPO}_3^{2-} \\
\| \\
\text{CH}_2
\end{array}
\quad
\xrightarrow[\text{pyruvate kinase}]{\text{ADP} \searrow \text{Mg}^{2+} \nearrow \text{ATP}}
\quad
\begin{array}{c}
\text{CO}\bar{\text{O}} \\
| \\
\text{C}=\text{O} \\
| \\
\text{CH}_3
\end{array}
$$

phosphoenolpyruvate   pyruvate

The reaction is highly exergonic and greatly favours pyruvate formation. Pyruvate kinases from higher plants are inhibited by citrate, ATP and calcium and have a requirement for magnesium and monovalent cations, notably potassium. However the amounts of citrate and ATP required are high and it may be that these compounds are not regulatory *in vivo*.

Under aerobic conditions the pyruvate produced from glycolysis is converted to acetyl-CoA via pyruvate oxidase and enters the tricarboxylic acid cycle where it is oxidised to carbon dioxide and water. Phosphoenolpyruvate can also be removed from the glycolytic pathway and converted to oxaloacetate in a reaction catalysed by phosphoenolpyruvate carboxylase. This serves as a mechanism for topping up the tricarboxylic acid cycle in tissues where a supply of keto acids is required for amino acid synthesis.

Under anaerobic conditions the end-products of glycolysis appear to be more variable and may include ethanol, lactate and alanine. Their formation is primarily a consequence of increased NADH levels due to inhibition of the respiratory chain when a plant is short of oxygen. Of course aerial organs such as leaves and stems are unlikely to experience anaerobic conditions but decreased oxygen levels may be observed in most cells during flooding or in developing and germinating seeds when oxygen access may be limited by poorly permeable outer layers.

The products of fermentation may vary with the plant or the length of anoxia but the significance of such variation is unknown. Alcohol dehydrogenase, the terminal enzyme of alcoholic fermentation, has been demonstrated in many plant species and activity is similar to that of other glycolytic enzymes. In spite of this, ethanol production is normally very low but increases markedly following the onset of anaerobic conditions. The switch to ethanol production is thought to operate directly on pyruvate metabolism, that is on pyruvate dehydrogenase or pyruvate decarboxylase (Fig. 4.3).

One explanation is that under anaerobic conditions there is an initial accumulation of organic acids which cause a fall in cell pH.

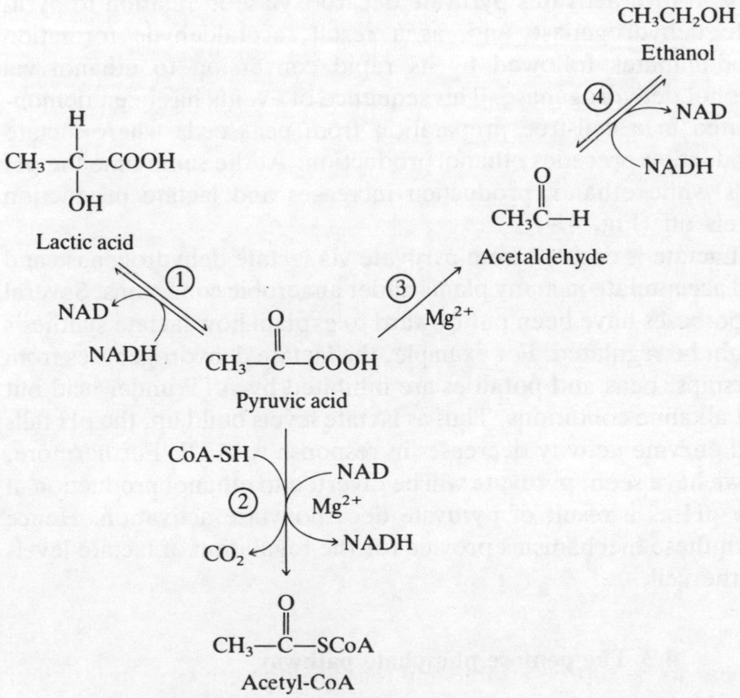

Fig. 4.3 Pyruvate metabolism.
(1) lactate dehydrogenase; (2) pyruvate dehydrogenase; (3) pyruvate decarboxylase; (4) alcohol dehydrogenase.

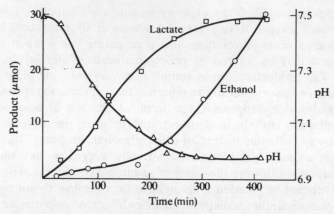

Fig. 4.4 Sequence of formation of lactate and ethanol in relation
to pH during glycolysis by an extract of pea seeds (From D. D.
Davies, S. Grego, and P. Kenworthy, 1974. *Planta* **118**, 297.)

This in turn activates pyruvate decarboxylase in relation to pyruvate dehydrogenase and, as a result, acetaldehyde formation predominates followed by its rapid conversion to ethanol via alcohol dehydrogenase. This sequence of events has been demonstrated in a cell-free preparation from pea seeds where lactate production precedes ethanol production. At the same time the pH falls while ethanol production increases and lactate production levels off (Fig. 4.4).

Lactate is derived from pyruvate via lactate dehydrogenase and can accumulate in many plants under anaerobic conditions. Several hypotheses have been put forward to explain how lactate synthesis might be regulated. For example, the lactate dehydrogenases from parsnips, peas and potatoes are inhibited by ATP under acid but not alkaline conditions. Thus as lactate levels build up, the pH falls and enzyme activity decreases in response to ATP. Furthermore, as we have seen, pyruvate will be diverted to ethanol production at low pH as a result of pyruvate decarboxylase activation. Hence both these mechanisms provide for the regulation of lactate levels in the cell.

4.3 The pentose phosphate pathway

In addition to glycolysis there exists a second pathway for the cellular oxidation of hexose phosphates. This is variously known as the pentose phosphate pathway (PPP) or hexose monophosphate shunt (Fig. 4.5). The overall reaction is essentially one in which glucose-6-phosphate is converted to fructose-6-phosphate and glyceraldehyde-3-phosphate.

In mammalian systems the PPP is active in tissues synthesizing fatty acids, such as adipose tissue and lactating mammary gland. One of its major functions, therefore, is considered to be the supply of reduced NADP for lipid synthesis. There is also direct evidence that the reduced NADP required for lignin synthesis comes from the PPP. Another important function may be the provision of pentose phosphate and erythrose phosphate for, the synthesis of nucleic acids and aromatic compounds respectively.

An alternative route for glucose metabolism was first suspected when it was shown that in some tissues glucose continued to be utilized in the presence of inhibitors of glycolysis such as iodoacetate and fluoride. Later work showed that this was accounted for by the operation of the PPP and it is now generally recognized that this operates in a wide range of living tissues including those of higher plants. The pathway differs from glycolysis in a number of ways: oxidation takes place in the first reactions with the production of reduced NADP, carbon dioxide is evolved and no energy is directly trapped.

The conversion of glucose-6-phosphate to the ketopentose ribulose-5-phosphate, sometimes referred to as the oxidative section of the PPP, is irreversible at the gluconolactone hydrolase step. The subsequent reactions in which ribulose-5-phosphate is converted to fructose-6-phosphate and glyceraldehyde-3-phosphate, sometimes referred to as the non-oxidative section of the pathway, are readily reversible. Since many of the enzymes involved have wide specificity, the exact reactions involved cannot be specified with confidence. Thus, although the overall sequence of reactions shown in Fig. 4.5 is generally agreed, some slight deviation is always possible.

4.3.1 Fate of products

These may be metabolized in a number of ways. The fructose-6-phosphate may be recycled in the PPP following conversion to glucose-6-phosphate; it may be converted to glucose-1-phosphate and then enter the pathways of sucrose and polysaccharide synthesis; or it may be metabolized in the glycolytic pathway. In those parts of the plant which have significant fructose-1,6-bisphosphatase activity, such as photosynthetic tissues, the

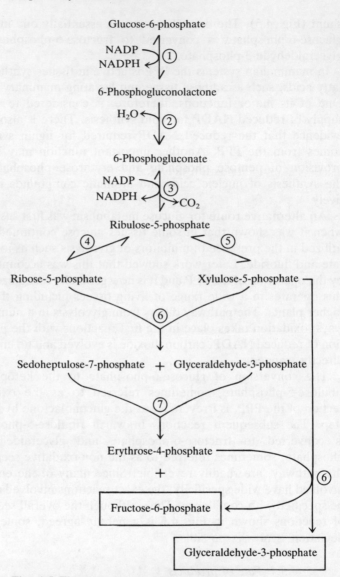

Fig. 4.5 The pentose phosphate pathway.
(1) glucose-6-phosphate dehydrogenase; (2) gluconolactone
hydrolase; (3) 6-phosphogluconate dehydrogenase; (4) ribose
phosphate isomerase; (5) ribulose-5-phosphate epimerase;
(6) transketolase; (7) transaldolase.

glyceraldehyde-3-phosphate may be converted to fructose-6-phosphate in a reaction sequence catalysed by aldolase and fructose-1,6-bisphosphatase. This in turn may then be converted to polysaccharide (§5.1) or recycled through the PPP. In non-photosynthetic tissues, however, the glyceraldehyde-3-phosphate most likely will enter the pool of glycolytic intermediates and be metabolized to pyruvate and other respiratory products.

4.3.2 Control mechanisms

It seems likely that flux through the PPP is regulated by the activity of glucose-6-phosphate dehydrogenase. This enzyme is inhibited by NADPH and activity seems to be controlled by the $NADP^+:NADPH$ ratio. Under conditions in which NADPH is oxidized, flux through the PPP increases, presumably as a result of decreased inhibition of glucose-6-phosphate dehydrogenase. Further work suggests that changes in dehydrogenase activity may be correlated with stage of tissue development. For example, activity increases markedly during endosperm development in barley. This may be associated with an increased supply of pentose phosphates required for nucleic acid and nucleotide synthesis at this stage of endosperm development. In other tissues, such as differentiating pea roots, there is evidence (ap Rees, 1980a) to suggest that the changes in enzyme activity are related to changes in flux through the PPP.

4.4 Glycolysis and the pentose phosphate pathway

Clearly there is a close relationship between the two pathways since they have a number of enzymes and intermediates in common. It seems likely that the two almost always operate together and the products of the PPP may, under certain conditions, be metabolized via the glycolytic pathway. Before the general pattern of carbohydrate metabolism in plants can be fully understood the relative contribution of each of these pathways to overall carbohydrate oxidation should be assessed. Much of the recent progress in this area has been made by ap Rees and his colleagues.

4.4.1 Localization of glycolysis and the pentose phosphate pathway

The enzymes of both pathways are soluble in the cytosol. However, there is evidence to suggest that some are also present in chloroplasts and some proplastids. Several of the enzymes of the photosynthetic carbon reduction cycle are held in common with both glycolysis and the PPP. Those which would be required to give a full complement of PPP enzymes are glucose-6-phosphate dehydrogenase, 6-phosphogluconate dehydrogenase, transaldolase and phosphofructokinase. These have been shown to be present in chloroplasts. Thus if these enzymes are used in conjunction with those of the photosynthetic carbon reduction cycle, chloroplasts may then be capable of catalysing the complete PPP as well as glycolysis, at least as far as 3-phosphoglycerate. It seems likely that these pathways operate in the dark to degrade hexose phosphates, derived from starch hydrolysis, to triose phosphate and 3-phosphoglycerate.

These could then leave the chloroplast via the phosphate translocator. Thus this would provide a mechanism whereby carbohydrate synthesized in the light can be degraded subsequently in the dark, and the products used elsewhere for the maintenance of essential processes. It is also likely that some of the enzymes of glycolysis and the PPP are present in proplastids. In developing castor bean endosperm these are the site of fatty acid synthesis and it may be that some of the intermediates and energy required may originate within the proplastids themselves.

4.4.2 Measurement of the relative activities of glycolysis and pentose phosphate pathway

Most measurements have been carried out on non-photosynthetic tissues in order to avoid the extra complications posed by the presence of photorespiration (§4.7) and photosynthetic carbon dioxide fixation. Tissues used include roots and tubers, germinating seeds and the spadix of *Arum maculatum*. The simplest and most convenient method for assessing the relative contributions of the two pathways is to measure the $^{14}CO_2$ evolved from tissues fed with specifically labelled [^{14}C]hexoses. For example, in the PPP, carbon atom number 1 (C-1) of glucose is released first as CO_2 (Fig. 4.6), carbon atom number 6 (C-6) only being released later following further metabolism or recycling. In glycolysis, on the other hand C-1 and C-6 of the original glucose are both released as CO_2 following pyruvate oxidation. This is because triose phosphates, labelled in both C-1 and C-3 positions and derived from fructose-1,6-bisphosphate following aldolase action, equilibrate in a reaction catalysed by triose phosphate isomerase. Both C-1 and C-6 of the original glucose thus end up as the methyl group, or C_3,

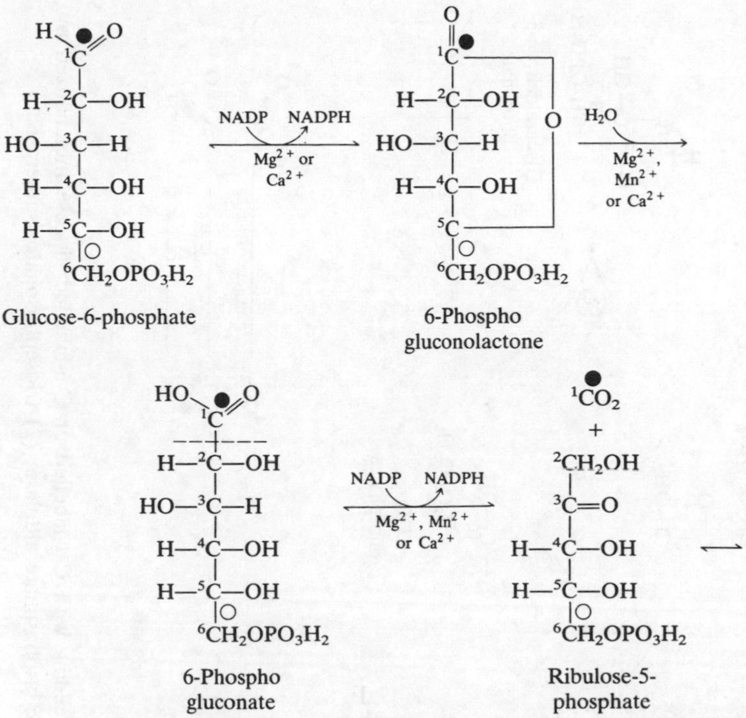

Fig. 4.6 Labelling of evolved carbon dioxide following feeding with C-1-labelled or C-6 labelled glucose metabolized by the pentose phosphate pathway.

of pyruvate (Fig. 4.7). When pyruvate is subsequently oxidized in the tricarboxylic acid cycle this would be the last CO_2 released. Hence by feeding replicate samples of tissue with glucose labelled in the C-1 and C-6 positions one might obtain an estimate for the contribution to glucose oxidation of each pathway by measuring the relative amounts of $^{14}CO_2$ evolved from ^{14}C-6-labelled and ^{14}C-1-labelled glucose respectively. This is referred to as the C-6:C-1 ratio. If glucose oxidation is solely via the PPP then the ratio should be zero since C-1 only is released. If intermediates are recycled then it will increase as C-6 is released. If glycolysis is the major pathway then the ratio will be 1.0 since both carbons are incorporated in the methyl group of pyruvate and the rates of release of $^{14}CO_2$ from C-1 and C-6 will be the same. If both pathways are operating simultaneously then the ratio will decrease as the contribution of the PPP increases.

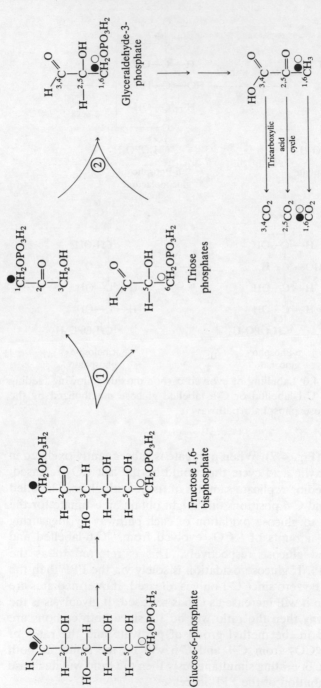

Fig. 4.7 Labelling of evolved carbon dioxide following feeding with C-1-labelled or C-6-labelled glucose metabolized by glycolysis and the tricarboxylic acid cycle. (1) fructose-1,6-bisphosphate aldolase; (2) triosephosphate isomerase.

Unfortunately although this method is relatively simple to carry out, it is generally agreed that in practice C-6:C-1 ratios cannot set a precise value for the contribution of each pathway. This is largely because cells do not operate the two pathways independently and in total isolation from other metabolic processes. Complications chiefly arise from recycling in the PPP and from the removal of intermediates, such as triose phosphate in other biochemical pathways. For example depending on whether the glucose fed is labelled in either the C-1- or C-6- position, recycling of pentose can change the labelling pattern and hence the specific activity of regenerated glucose-6-phosphate. That is [^{14}C-1] glucose metabolised in the pentose phosphate pathway, when recycled via pentose phosphate will give unlabelled glucose-6-phosphate, whereas [^{14}C-6] glucose-6-phosphate, when recycled will retain its original labelling pattern. Hence the C-6:C-1 ratio will increase as recycling continues. Obviously the degree of recycling will depend on the competition for hexose phosphate between the two pathways and on the removal of intermediates for biosynthesis. Such effects might be minimized by using excess glucose to reduce the relative amounts of recycled glucose, and by measuring ratios within a short time of glucose feeding.

In addition to problems caused by recycling, hexose labelling patterns will be complicated by the conversion of any triose phosphate intermediates to such products as amino acids or organic acids, and of hexose phosphates to sucrose or polysaccharides. Hence again the C-6: C-1 ratios will fail to give a satisfactory estimate of the relative activities of the two pathways.

More serious problems arise from the realisation that both pathways probably operate simultaneously and independently in the cytosol and the plastid. Thus the determinations described above only give an overall estimate of relative activities and do not strictly relate to the situation *in vivo*.

It is clear however, that both pathways are present in most plant tissues and that under most conditions the overall contribution of the PPP does not exceed 30 per cent of the total carbohydrate oxidised.

4.5 The tricarboxylic acid cycle

Most of the pyruvate derived from glycolysis and the PPP is metabolized in the tricarboxylic acid cycle. This was first described by Krebs and Johnson in 1937 working with pigeon breast muscle.

Subsequently it has been shown that the cycle operates almost universally in plants under aerobic conditions.

The enzymes of the cycle (Fig. 1.9) are located in the innermost compartment of the mitochondrion, the matrix, and the enzymes associated with electron transport and oxidative phosphorylation are located in the inner mitochondrial membrane. The pyruvate enters the mitochondria from the cytosol and is first converted to acetyl-CoA in a multistep reaction sequence catalysed by pyruvate dehydrogenase, lipoate acetyltransferase and dihydrolipoyl dehydrogenase (pyruvate dehydrogenase complex):

$$
\begin{array}{c}
COO \\
| \\
C=O \\
| \\
CH_3
\end{array}
\quad
\xrightarrow[\substack{\\ CoASH}]{\substack{CO_2 \qquad\qquad NAD \quad NADH \\ Mg^{2+}}}
\quad
\begin{array}{c}
O \\
\diagdown\!\!\!\diagup \\
C-SCoA \\
| \\
CH_3
\end{array}
$$

pyruvate   Thiamine pyrophosphate/lipoic acid   acetyl-CoA

pyruvate dehydrogenase complex

Decarboxylation is catalysed in a magnesium-dependent reaction through combination of the remaining two carbons with thiamine pyrophosphate. The two-carbon group is then transferred to lipoic acid and oxidized to an acetyl group. Finally this is transferred to CoA with the formation of acetyl-CoA. The oxidized lipoate is regenerated by dihydrolipoate dehydrogenase in a reaction where electrons are transferred from FAD with the eventual formation of NADH. The overall reaction is irreversible and it is likely that this is a site of regulation. The plant enzyme is inhibited by both acetyl-CoA and ATP but the concentrations required are high and it is unlikely that these act *in vivo* to regulate enzyme activity. On the other hand NADH strongly inhibits activity and this may be the means by which regulation is achieved.

Citrate synthase then catalyses the irreversible formation of citrate from acetyl-CoA and the acceptor oxaloacetate:

$$
\begin{array}{c}
CO\bar{O} \\
| \\
C=O \\
| \\
CH_2 \\
| \\
CO\bar{O}
\end{array}
+
\begin{array}{c}
O \\
\diagdown\!\!\!\diagup \\
C-SCoA \\
| \\
CH_3
\end{array}
\xrightarrow{\text{citrate synthase}}
\begin{array}{c}
COO \\
| \\
CH_2 \\
| \\
\bar{O}OC-C-OH + CoASH \\
| \\
CH_2 \\
| \\
CO\bar{O}
\end{array}
$$

oxaloacetate   acetyl-CoA   citrate

A reversible dehydration followed by hydration catalysed by aconitase gives rise to *cis*-aconitate and isocitrate:

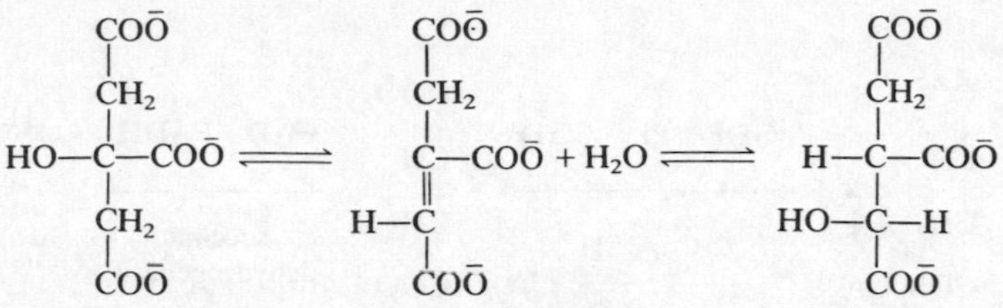

$$
\begin{array}{ccc}
\underset{\text{citrate}}{
\begin{array}{c}
COO^- \\
| \\
CH_2 \\
| \\
HO-C-COO^- \\
| \\
CH_2 \\
| \\
COO^-
\end{array}}
\rightleftharpoons
\underset{\text{\textit{cis}-aconitate}}{
\begin{array}{c}
COO^- \\
| \\
CH_2 \\
| \\
C-COO^- \quad + H_2O \\
\| \\
H-C \\
| \\
COO^-
\end{array}}
\rightleftharpoons
\underset{\text{isocitrate}}{
\begin{array}{c}
COO^- \\
| \\
CH_2 \\
| \\
H-C-COO^- \\
| \\
HO-C-H \\
| \\
COO^-
\end{array}}
\end{array}
$$

The formation of α-ketoglutarate is catalysed by isocitrate dehydrogenase in a decarboxylation reaction dependent on magnesium or manganese ions:

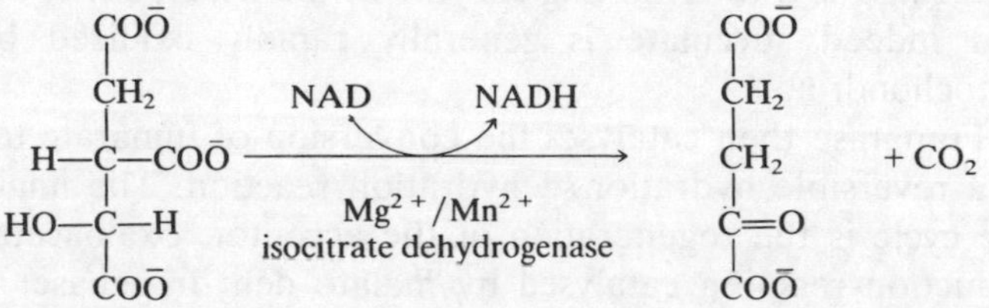

$$
\underset{\text{isocitrate}}{
\begin{array}{c}
COO^- \\
| \\
CH_2 \\
| \\
H-C-COO^- \\
| \\
HO-C-H \\
| \\
COO^-
\end{array}}
\xrightarrow[\substack{Mg^{2+}/Mn^{2+} \\ \text{isocitrate dehydrogenase}}]{\quad NAD \quad NADH \quad}
\underset{\alpha\text{-ketoglutarate}}{
\begin{array}{c}
COO^- \\
| \\
CH_2 \\
| \\
CH_2 \quad + CO_2 \\
| \\
C=O \\
| \\
COO^-
\end{array}}
$$

The next reaction of the tricarboxylic acid cycle is the oxidation of α-ketoglutarate by NAD, accompanied by decarboxylation. The remaining four-carbon unit forms the thiol ester, succinyl-CoA. The overall reaction is irreversible:

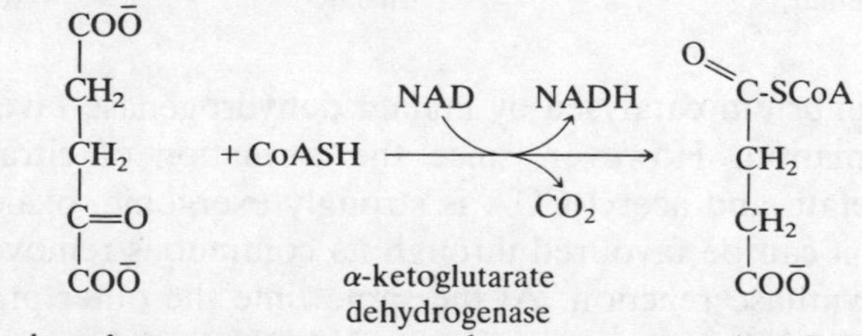

$$
\underset{\alpha\text{-ketoglutarate}}{
\begin{array}{c}
COO^- \\
| \\
CH_2 \\
| \\
CH_2 \quad + CoASH \\
| \\
C=O \\
| \\
COO^-
\end{array}}
\xrightarrow[\substack{\alpha\text{-ketoglutarate} \\ \text{dehydrogenase} \\ \text{complex}}]{\quad NAD \quad NADH \quad CO_2}
\underset{\text{succinyl-CoA}}{
\begin{array}{c}
\overset{O}{\underset{\|}{C}}\text{-SCoA} \\
| \\
CH_2 \\
| \\
CH_2 \\
| \\
COO^-
\end{array}}
$$

The conversion of succinyl-CoA to succinate, catalysed by succinyl-CoA synthetase, is highly exergonic and the energy released is used to synthesize a nucleoside triphosphate, probably adenosine triphosphate. The conversion of succinate to fumarate is catalysed by succinate dehydrogenase, an enzyme tightly bound to the mitochondrial membrane and, therefore, often used as a convenient marker for mitochondrial activity:

$$
\begin{array}{c}
CO\bar{O} \\
| \\
CH_2 \\
| \\
CH_2 \\
| \\
COSCoA
\end{array}
\quad
\xrightarrow[\substack{\text{CoA-SH} \\ \text{succinyl-CoA} \\ \text{synthetase}}]{\substack{\text{GDP + Pi} \quad \text{GTP}}}
\quad
\begin{array}{c}
CO\bar{O} \\
| \\
CH_2 \\
| \\
CH_2 \\
| \\
CO\bar{O}
\end{array}
\quad
\xrightarrow[\text{dehydrogenase}]{\substack{\text{FAD} \quad \text{FADH} \\ \text{succinic}}}
\quad
\begin{array}{c}
H \qquad CO\bar{O} \\
\diagdown \quad \diagup \\
C \\
\| \\
C \\
\diagup \quad \diagdown \\
\bar{O}OC \qquad H
\end{array}
$$

succinyl-CoA   succinate   fumarate

Succinic dehydrogenase is activated by a number of cell metabolites including ATP and succinyl-CoA, and strongly inhibited by oxaloacetate. However, there is no evidence that succinic dehydrogenase is a rate-limiting enzyme in the tricarboxylic acid cycle and indeed succinate is generally rapidly oxidized by plant mitochondria.

Fumarase then catalyses the conversion of fumarate to malate in a reversible hydration/dehydration reaction. The final step of the cycle is the regeneration of the acceptor, oxaloacetate, in a reduction reaction catalysed by malate dehydrogenase:

$$
\begin{array}{c}
H \qquad COOH \\
\diagdown \quad \diagup \\
C \\
\| \\
C \\
\diagup \quad \diagdown \\
\bar{H}OOC \qquad H
\end{array}
\quad + H_2O \rightleftharpoons[\text{fumarase}]{}
\quad
\begin{array}{c}
CO\bar{O} \\
| \\
HOCH \\
| \\
CH_2 \\
| \\
CO\bar{O}
\end{array}
\quad
\xrightleftharpoons[\text{dehydrogenase}]{\substack{\text{NAD} \quad \text{NADH} \\ \text{malate}}}
\quad
\begin{array}{c}
CO\bar{O} \\
| \\
C{=}O \\
| \\
CH_2 \\
| \\
CO\bar{O}
\end{array}
$$

fumarate   malate   oxaloacetate

The equilibrium catalysed by malate dehydrogenase favours malate formation. However, since the formation of citrate from oxaloacetate and acetyl-COA is strongly exergonic, oxaloacetate formation can be favoured through its continuous removal in the citrate synthase reaction. At the same time the other product of the malate dehydrogenase reaction, NADH, may be removed by oxidation via the electron transfer chain. Other mechanisms may also contribute to the displacement of the malate dehydrogenase equilibrium. For example, in cells active in the biosynthesis of amino acids some oxaloacetate will be removed from the cycle during transamination with glutamate.

Additionally malate itself may be removed in a decarboxylation reaction catalysed by malic enzyme:

$$\underset{\text{malate}}{\begin{array}{c} \overline{COO} \\ | \\ HO-CH \\ | \\ CH_2 \\ | \\ \overline{COO} \end{array}} \quad \overset{NAD \qquad NADH}{\underset{\text{malic enzyme}}{\overset{Mn^{2+}}{\rightleftharpoons}}} \quad \underset{\text{pyruvate}}{\begin{array}{c} \overline{COO} \\ | \\ C=O \\ | \\ CH_3 \end{array}} + CO_2$$

This reaction is reversible and present in most plant mitochondria. One of the possible fates of the pyruvate formed may be conversion to acetyl-CoA in the pyruvate dehydrogenase reaction. The acetyl-CoA may then re-enter the tricarboxylic acid cycle following combination with oxaloacetate in the citrate synthase reaction (Palmer, 1976). Effectively this means that acetyl-CoA can be

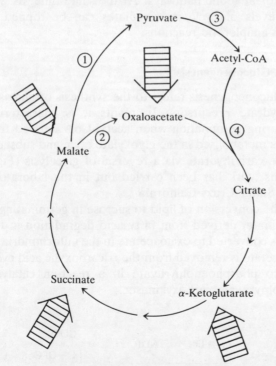

Fig. 4.8 Regeneration of acetyl-CoA from externally supplied intermediates of the tricarboxylic acid cycle. (1) malic enzyme; (2) malate dehydrogenase; (3) pyruvate dehydrogenase; (4) citrate synthase.

regenerated from cycle intermediates. Thus a mechanism exists whereby intermediates may be fed into the cycle and oxidized without the need for external supplies of acetyl-CoA (Fig. 4.8).

Such intermediates may include oxaloacetate, α-ketoglutarate, malate and succinate. Both oxaloacetate and α-ketoglutarate may be derived from pathways of amino acid metabolism following transamination reactions. Oxaloacetate and malate may be derived from glycolysis following conversion of phosphoenolpyruvate to malate via cytoplasmic phosphoenolpyruvate carboxylase and NADP malate dehydrogenase. Following uptake by the mitochondrion, malate may enter the tricarboxylic acid cycle. Succinate formed from fatty acid degradation in the glyoxysomes may also be oxidized by the tricarboxylic acid cycle.

Thus the tricarboxylic acid cycle functions not only in the direct oxidation of pyruvate from glycolysis but also in the provision of precursors for anabolic pathways. At the same time, as we have seen, the levels of cycle intermediates can be topped up by auxiliary or anaplerotic reactions.

4.6 Gluconeogenesis

The term gluconeogenesis refers to the synthesis of glucose from non-carbohydrate precursors. In plants it is characteristically observed during germination when acetyl-CoA derived from reserve lipid is metabolised in the glyoxylate cycle and subsequently converted to carbohydrate via a reversal of glycolysis (Fig. 3.3). Much of this work has been carried out in the laboratories of Beevers at Santa Cruz, California.

During the conversion of lipid to sucrose in germinating castor beans, succinate, derived from fatty acid degradation in the glyoxysomes, is converted to oxaloacetate in the mitochondria (§3.4). The oxaloacetate is removed from the tricarboxylic acid cycle and converted to phosphoenolpyruvate in a reaction catalysed by phosphoenolpyruvate carboxykinase:

$$
\begin{array}{l}
\overset{|}{C}OO^{\bar{}} \\
\overset{|}{C}{=}O \\
\overset{|}{C}H_2 \\
\overset{|}{C}OO^{\bar{}}
\end{array}
\quad
\xrightarrow[\substack{\text{phosphoenolpyruvate} \\ \text{carboxykinase}}]{\text{ATP} \qquad \text{ADP}}
\quad
\begin{array}{l}
\overset{|}{C}OO^{\bar{}} \\
\overset{\|}{C}{-}OPO_3^{2-} \quad +\, CO_2 \\
CH_2
\end{array}
$$

oxaloacetate   phosphoenolpyruvate

Enzyme activity increases during marrow seed germination and correlates well with overall rates of gluconeogenesis. The phosphoenolpyruvate may then be converted to fructose-1,6-bisphosphate via the reversible reactions of glycolysis (Fig. 4.2). The phosphofructokinase reaction may then be .bypassed by the conversion of fructose-1,6-bisphosphate to fructose-6-phosphate in a reaction catalysed by fructose-1,6-bisphosphatase.

$$\text{D-fructose-1,6-bisphosphate} + H_2O \longrightarrow$$
$$\text{D-fructose-6-phosphate} + H_3PO_4$$

Again activity increased markedly during marrow seed germination. In germinating castor bean seeds the activity of both these gluconeogenic enzymes is sufficient to account for the observed rates of gluconeogenesis which are up to 10 times the rate of glycolysis.

The two pathways of glycolysis and gluconeogenesis are presumably regulated independently so that both do not operate simultaneously. In marrow cotyledons, evidence that both phosphoenolpyruvate carboxylase and fructose-1,6-bisphosphatase might be regulatory enzymes comes from work showing increased levels of their substrates, oxaloacetate and fructose-1,6-bisphosphate, when gluconeogenesis is inhibited with 3-mercaptopicolinic acid. However, since this tissue contains both phosphoenolpyruvate carboxylase and phosphofructokinase activity the observed increases could be due to changes in activity of these two glycolytic enzymes rather than in the activity of phosphoenolpyruvate carboxykinase and fructose-1,6-bisphosphatase. One key to the regulation of the two pathways may lie in the fact that fructose-1,6-bisphosphatase is inhibited by AMP. Thus since gluconeogenesis in marrow cotyledons is accompanied by an increase in ATP levels as a result of β-oxidation, and an associated decrease in AMP levels, inhibition of the bisphosphatase should be relieved during germination (ap Rees, 1980b). Additionally, maximum catalytic activity of the equivalent glycolytic enzyme, phosphofructokinase, is less than 5 per cent of that of fructose-1,6-bisphosphatase. Thus gluconeogenesis should be favoured under these conditions (see also §8.3).

Differential regulation of glycolysis and gluconeogenesis may also be exerted at the level of phosphoenolpyruvate metabolism. During gluconeogenesis, oxaloacetate is converted to fructose-6-phosphate via phosphoenolpyruvate. The competing reaction of glycolysis is the conversion of phosphoenolpyruvate to pyruvate in the reaction catalysed by pyruvate kinase. If, as seems possible, pyruvate kinase is inhibited by ATP, the conversion of phosphoenolpyruvate to pyruvate will be prevented during gluconeogenesis due to the increased levels of ATP. These mechanisms can then ensure that the two pathways do not complete directly in a futile cycle for the same substrates.

4.7 Photorespiration and glycolate metabolism

The oxygen uptake and associated carbon dioxide formation directly due to the effect of light on photosynthetic metabolism is called photorespiration. Evidence for a light-stimulated evolution of carbon dioxide comes from experiments in which carbon dioxide-free air is rapidly swept over illuminated leaves. The rate of carbon dioxide fixation is decreased by the absence of substrate and carbon dioxide release into the air stream can be detected. In some plants, this release is higher in the light than in the dark. In other species no light-stimulated release of carbon dioxide can be measured.

Further evidence for the existence of photorespiration is based on the observation that there is a rapid evolution of carbon dioxide following darkening. This is called the post-illumination carbon dioxide burst. In tobacco leaves it rises to a brief maximum value and falls to the lower steady state within about 40s of turning off the light (Fig. 4.9). Thus, although photosynthesis ceases immediately

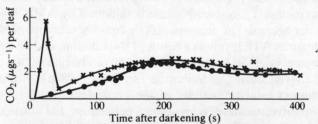

Fig. 4.9 The carbon dioxide burst observed in darkness following illumination of a detached tobacco leaf (*Nicotiana tabacum* L.). (From E. B. Tregunna, G. Krotkov, and C. D. Nelson, 1966. *Physiol. Plant.* **19**, 723.)

×   21 per cent oxygen;

•   2 per cent oxygen.

the light is turned off it seems that photorespiration runs on a little longer, resulting in a gush of carbon dioxide. This suggests that the substrate for photorespiration is synthesized in the light and that the carbon dioxide burst is a result of its further metabolism, normally obscured by carbon dioxide fixation in the light. The burst is not observed at low levels of oxygen, suggesting that oxygen is required for synthesis of the photorespiratory substrate. At the same time photosynthesis is inhibited by oxygen. Carbon dioxide has the opposite effect, in that it has an inhibitory effect on photorespiration but a stimulatory effect on photosynthesis. Thus, it seems likely that the balance between photorespiration and photosynthesis can be regulated by variation in carbon dioxide and oxygen levels.

4.7.1 Glycolate synthesis

It is now considered that the carbon dioxide evolved during photorespiration is produced as a result of glycolate metabolism. Glycolate itself is derived from phosphoglycolate, which in turn is the product of ribulose-1,5-bisphosphate oxygenation during photosynthesis. Evidence for the origin of glycolate comes from a number of different types of experiment. For example, from studies of the time course of incorporation of ^{14}C-labelled carbon dioxide into photosynthetic products by intact isolated chloroplasts, it is clear that glycolate is labelled only after intermediates of the photosynthetic carbon reduction cycle have become labelled. It is, therefore, likely that glycolate is derived from one or more sugar phosphate intermediates of the carbon reduction cycle. Further evidence comes from experiments in which sugar phosphates are supplied to intact chloroplasts. Thus, it was shown using inhibitors of photophosphorylation, that glycolate formation from triose or pentose monophosphates is ATP-dependent. It is unlikely, therefore, that glycolate is derived from an intermediate of the reaction sequence between triose phosphate and ribulose-5-phosphate since none of these reactions requires ATP. The formation of ribulose-1,5-bisphosphate from ribulose-5-phosphate requires ATP and it is probable that glycolate is formed directly from ribulose-1,5-bisphosphate (Krause *et al.*, 1977). The formation of phosphoglycolate in the reaction catalysed by ribulose-1,5-bisphosphate carboxylase–oxygenase appears to be the major route of glycolate formation. The products are equimolar amounts of phosphoglycolate and phosphoglyceric acid:

$$
\begin{array}{ccc}
\underset{\text{ribulose-1,5-bisphosphate}}{
\begin{array}{c}
\text{CH}_2\text{OPO}_3^{2-} \\
| \\
\text{C}{=}\text{O} \\
| \\
\text{H}{-}\text{C}{-}\text{OH} \\
| \\
\text{H}{-}\text{C}{-}\text{OH} \\
| \\
\text{CH}_2\text{OPO}_3^{2-}
\end{array}}
&
\xrightarrow[\substack{\text{ribulose-1,5-bisphosphate} \\ \text{carboxylase–oxygenase}}]{\text{O}_2}
&
\begin{array}{l}
\begin{array}{c}
\text{CH}_2\text{OPO}_3^{2-} \\
| \\
\text{CO\={O}}
\end{array} \\
\text{phosphoglycolate} \\[4pt]
\underset{\text{phosphoglyceric acid}}{
\begin{array}{c}
\text{CO\={O}} \\
| \\
\text{H}{-}\text{C}{-}\text{OH} \\
| \\
\text{CH}_2\text{OPO}_3^{2-}
\end{array}}
\end{array}
\end{array}
$$

A specific phosphoglycolate phosphatase, localised in the chloroplast, then catalyses the formation of glycolate from phosphoglycolate:

$$
\underset{\text{phosphoglycolate}}{
\begin{array}{c}
\text{CH}_2\text{OPO}_3^{2-} \\
| \\
\text{CO\={O}}
\end{array}}
\xrightarrow[\text{phosphatase}]{\text{phosphoglycolate}}
\underset{\text{glycolate}}{
\begin{array}{c}
\text{CH}_2\text{OH} \\
| \\
\text{CO\={O}H}
\end{array}}
$$

The properties of ribulose-1,5-bisphosphate carboxylase–oxygenase suggest an explanation for the differential effects of oxygen and carbon dioxide on photosynthesis and photorespiration. That is, carboxylating activity is inhibited competitively by oxygen when carbon dioxide is a substrate and oxygenase activity is inhibited competitively by carbon dioxide when oxgyen is a substrate. Thus, photosynthetic carbon dioxide fixation is inhibited by oxygen and promoted by carbon dioxide. Similarly, glycolate formation, or photorespiration, is inhibited by carbon dioxide and promoted by oxygen. Oxygenase activity increases relative to the carboxylase activity with increasing temperature. Hence at elevated temperatures, photorespiration will increase relative to photosynthesis.

4.7.2 Glycolate metabolism
Glycolate metabolism involves the co-operation of chloroplasts, cytosol, peroxisomes and mitochondria since the enzymes involved are distributed among these cell compartments. Glycolate synthesized in the chloroplast is thought to enter the peroxisome where it is first converted to glyoxylate in a reaction catalysed by glycolate oxidase (Fig. 4.10). This enzyme has a low affinity for oxygen, again suggesting a reason for the stimulation of photorespiration by oxygen. The hydrogen peroxide released is converted to water and oxygen by peroxisomal catalase. Thus the net oxygen

uptake during the oxidation of one molecule of glycolate is half a molecule of oxygen. In a second peroxisomal reaction glyoxylate is converted to glycine in a transaminase reaction where the amino donor can be glutamate or serine. The glycine then moves to the mitochondrion where it is converted to serine and carbon dioxide by glycine decarboxylase and serine hydroxymethyl transferase. Two molecules of glycine are required for the synthesis of one molecule of serine. Following transfer to the peroxisome the serine is converted to hydroxypyruvate and then glycerate in two reactions catalysed by a transaminase and hydroxypyruvate reductase respectively. Finally the glycerate enters the chloroplast where it is phosphorylated to form phosphoglyceric acid.

The major source of photorespiratory carbon dioxide is the reaction in which glycine is converted to serine. *In vivo* turnover rates of glycine are apparently sufficient to produce carbon dioxide at rates equivalent to those released in photorespiration. In addition to releasing carbon dioxide the glycine decarboxylase reaction generates an equivalent amount of ammonia. Since the rate of photorespiration is greater than that of nitrate assimilation it is assumed that a proportion of the ammonia released (if not all) is refixed, since otherwise the plant would lose much of its protein.

The overall effect of glycolate synthesis and metabolism may be seen as the regeneration of phosphoglycerate from ribulose-1,5-bisphosphate. This process requires the input of energy and reducing power, whereas the direct conversion of ribulose-1,5-bisphosphate to phosphoglycerate via ribulose-1,5-bisphosphate carboxylase does not. Furthermore, between one-half and one-sixth of the carbon fixed in photosynthesis can be lost via photorespiration in C_3 plants. The failure to measure release of photorespiratory carbon dioxide in C_4 plants may be due to a reduction in the occurrence of photorespiration caused by increased levels of carbon dioxide in the bundle sheath cells as well as refixation of any carbon dioxide released.

The possible benefit, if any, to the plant of photorespiratory metabolism has been subject to much speculation. One possibility is that photorespiratory energy consumption may protect plants from damage due to overaccumulation of photochemical energy. Another possibility is that oxygenation is an unavoidable side reaction to carboxylation and that the photorespiratory conversion of phosphoglycolate back to phosphoglycerate is a mechanism for recovering at least 75 per cent of the carbon lost from the photosynthetic carbon reduction cycle.

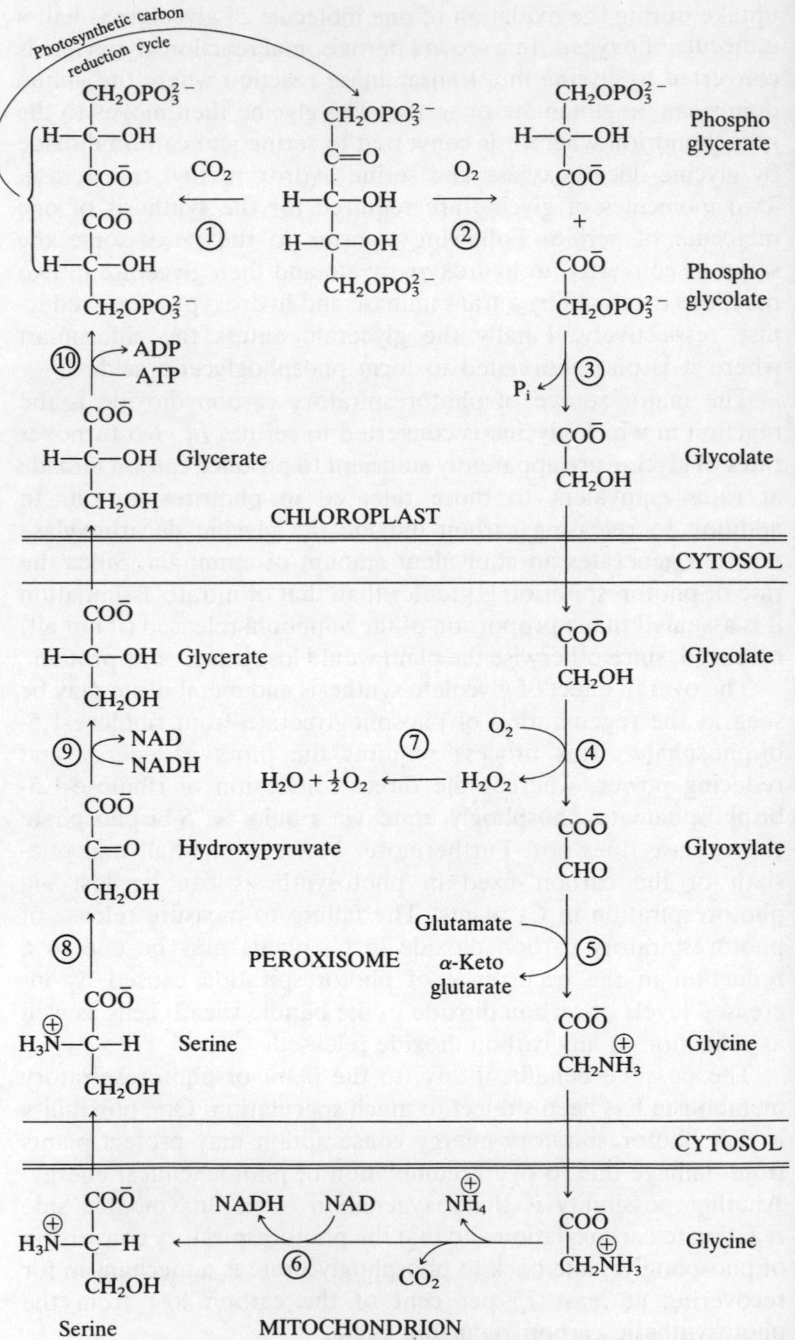

Photosynthetic carbon reduction cycle

$CH_2OPO_3^{2-}$
H—C—OH
COO⁻

COO⁻
H—C—OH
$CH_2OPO_3^{2-}$

$CH_2OPO_3^{2-}$
C=O
H—C—OH
H—C—OH
$CH_2OPO_3^{2-}$

CO_2 ①   ←   →   ② O_2

$CH_2OPO_3^{2-}$
H—C—OH
COO⁻   Phospho glycerate

+

COO⁻
$CH_2OPO_3^{2-}$ Phospho glycolate

⑩ ⤵ ADP
      ATP

COO⁻
H—C—OH   Glycerate
CH_2OH

③ P_i

COO⁻
CH_2OH Glycolate

CHLOROPLAST

CYTOSOL

COO⁻
H—C—OH   Glycerate
CH_2OH

COO⁻
CH_2OH Glycolate

⑨ ⤵ NAD
      NADH

⑦ $H_2O + \frac{1}{2}O_2$ ← H_2O_2 ← ④ O_2

COO⁻
C=O   Hydroxypyruvate
CH_2OH

COO⁻
CHO   Glyoxylate

⑧

PEROXISOME

Glutamate

α-Keto glutarate   ⑤

COO⁻
$H_3\overset{\oplus}{N}$—C—H   Serine
CH_2OH

COO⁻
$CH_2\overset{\oplus}{N}H_3$ Glycine

CYTOSOL

COO⁻
$H_3\overset{\oplus}{N}$—C—H
CH_2OH

NADH   NAD $\overset{\oplus}{N}H_4$

⑥

CO_2

COO⁻
$CH_2\overset{\oplus}{N}H_3$ Glycine

Serine   MITOCHONDRION

4.7.3 Photorespiration and 'dark' respiration

Although all respiratory activity in plants ultimately depends on photosynthesis, photorespiration is more closely dependent on the photosynthetic carbon dioxide reduction cycle than is 'dark' respiration since ribulose-1,5-bisphosphate is the immediate substrate. Thus photorespiration is found only in those cells active in photosynthetic carbon dioxide fixation whereas 'dark' respiration is characteristically present in most plant tissues. The most obvious point of contrast between the two types of respiration relates to their role in energy metabolism. The oxidation of carbohydrate, lipid and protein in 'dark' respiration provides energy and intermediates required for biosynthetic reactions. On the other hand, the oxygenation of ribulose-1,5-bisphosphate and the regeneration of phosphoglycerate via glycolate requires energy in the form of ATP and reducing equivalents. Any role of the intermediates of glycolate metabolism in the synthesis of photosynthetic end-products is thought to be a minor one. The common feature of both types of respiration is, of course, the consumption of oxygen and evolution of carbon dioxide.

References

ap Rees, T. (1980a) Assessment of the contributions of metabolic pathways to plant respiration, in *The Biochemistry of Plants,* Vol. 2. (P. K. Stumpf and E. E. Conn, eds.) Academic Press: New York.

ap Rees, T. (1980b) Integration of pathways of synthesis and degradation of hexose phosphates, in *The Biochemistry of Plants*. Vol. 3. (P. K. Stumpf and E. E. Conn, eds.) Academic Press: New York.

Davies, D. D. (1980) Aerobic metabolism and the production of organic acids, in *The Biochemistry of Plants*. Vol. 2. (P. K. Stumpf and E. E. Conn, eds.) Academic Press: New York.

Fig. 4.10 Glycolate synthesis and metabolism illustrating the role of chloroplasts, cytosol, peroxisomes and mitochondria.
(1) ribulose-1,5-bisphosphate carboxylase; (2) ribulose-1,5-bisphosphate oxygenase; (3) phosphoglycolate phosphatase; (4) glycolate oxidase; (5) glutamate-glyoxylate aminotransferase; (6) glycine decarboxylase and serine hydroxymethyl transferase; (7) catalase; (8) glutamate-hydroxypyruvate aminotransferase; (9) NADH-hydroxypruvate reductase or glycerate dehydrogenase; (10) glycerate kinase.

Krause, G. H., Thorne, S. W. and Lorimer, G. H. (1977)
Glycolate synthesis by intact chloroplasts, *Arch. Biochem. Biophys.* **183**, 471–9.

Lorimer, G. H. and Andrews, T. J. (1981) The C_2 chemo- and photorespiratory carbon oxidation cycle, in *The Biochemistry of Plants* Vol. 8. (P.K. Stumpf and E.E. Conn, eds.) (11) Academic Press: New York.

Opik, H. (1980) The Respiration of Higher Plants, (Studies in Biology No. 120). Edward Arnold.

Palmer, J. M. (1976) The organization and regulation of electron transport in plant mitochondria. *Ann. Rev. Plant Physiol.* **27**, 133–57.

Tolbert, N. E. (1979) Glycolate metabolism by higher plants and algae, in *Photosynthesis II Encyclopaedia of Plant Physiology (N.S.)*, Vol. 6. (M. Gibbs and E. Latzko, eds.) Springer-Verlag.

Turner, J. F. and Turner, D. H. (1980) The regulation of glycolysis and the pentose phosphate pathway, in *The Biochemistry of Plants*, Vol. 2. (P. K. Stumpf and E. E. Conn, eds.) Academic Press.

Wiskich, T. (1980) Control of the Krebs cycle, in *The Biochemistry of Plants*, Vol. 2. (P. K. Stumpf and E. E. Conn, eds.) Academic Press.

5

Polysaccharide synthesis

Polysaccharides can account for up to 85 per cent of plant dry weight and are the major yield component in agricultural crop production. Of these, starch is the dominating influence in world food production, largely because cereal grains, which contain 60–70 per cent starch, account for over half of our dietary energy supply. Apart from the food industry, starch products are also used in the textile, paper and pharmaceutical industries as well as in the offshore oil industry where they are present in the artificial muds used during the drilling of wells. Most of the remaining polysaccharide in higher plants is associated with the cell wall and, with the exception of cellulose and other β-D-glucans, consists of heteroglycans which fall into a limited number of structural groups (§2.3.2). Economically these are important as major constituents of woody tissues and pasture herbages. For example, the diet of grazing animals, on which many agricultural systems depend, consists largely of polysaccharide, mainly as cellulose and heteroglycans with some starch and fructan.

The mechanisms which may be involved in the control of polysaccharide synthesis in plants are of considerable interest. This is partly because they are fundamental to our understanding of plant cell growth and development. In addition, because of their enormous economic importance, it may be possible that, by identifying the biological limitations to polysaccharide synthesis, methods might be devised to modify these with the hope of increasing the amounts produced.

5.1 Origins of sugar nucleotide precursors

During polysaccharide synthesis the monosaccharide subunits are transferred from their nucleotide derivatives to the growing chain.

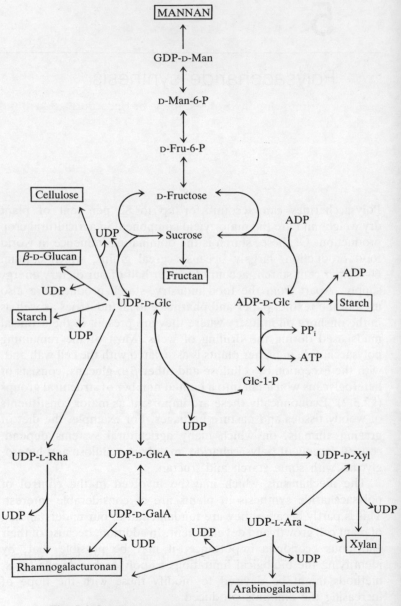

Fig. 5.1 Sucrose as a source of nucleotide sugar precursors used in the synthesis of polysaccharides.
Ara, arabinose; Fru, fructose; GalA, galacturonic acid; GDP, guanosine diphosphate; Glc, glucose; GlcA, glucuronic acid; Man, mannose; Rha, rhamnose; Xyl, xylose.

In turn, these nucleotide sugar precursors may be synthesized from sucrose and the corresponding nucleoside phosphate (Fig. 5.1). Sucrose, however, is not necessarily the direct source of polysaccharide precursors. Reserves may also be utilized in the synthesis of new polysaccharides. In germinating seeds and other tissues, monosaccharides, released from cell wall polysaccharides and starch following hydrolysis, may be incorporated without further modification into the nucleotide sugar pool and used directly in polysaccharide synthesis (Fig. 5.2).

Where polysaccharides are derived from sucrose, the key intermediate is probably UDP-glucose which serves as a direct precursor in the synthesis of cellulose, β-D-glucan and starch as well as of the sugar nucleotides, UDP-D-glucuronate, UDP-L-rhamnose, UDP-D-galacturonate, UDP-D-xylose, UDP-L-arabinose, etc. D-Fructose, released in the synthesis of UDP-glucose from sucrose in the reaction catalysed by sucrose synthase, may be used in the synthesis of GDP-mannose and also, after conversion to glucose-1-phosphate, in the synthesis of UDP-glucose (Fig. 5.1). UDP-glucose may also be derived from sucrose indirectly, following hydrolytic cleavage to glucose and fructose by the action of invertase (Fig. 5.2). Sucrose is also a direct precursor in the synthesis of fructan.

Where reserves are being used in the synthesis of new polysaccharide, the monosaccharides are first phosphorylated by ATP in a number of reactions catalysed by specific kinases (Fig. 5.2). Many of these are 1-kinases, that is the reaction results in the formation of monosaccharides phosphorylated at the C-1 position. These include L-arabinokinase and D-galacturonokinase.

On the other hand, D-glucose, D-fructose and D-mannose are phosphorylated in reactions catalysed by hexokinases which result in the formation of the 6-phospho derivatives. Isomerases may then convert fructose-6-phosphate to glucose-6-phosphate or mannose-6-phosphate and these, in turn, may be converted to glucose-1-phosphate or mannose-1-phosphate. Subsequently, the nucleotide sugars may be formed from the 1-phospho glycosyl derivatives and the respective nucleoside triphosphate in a reversible reaction catalysed by a pyrophosphorylase enzyme:

$$NTP + glycosyl\text{-}1\text{-}phosphate \rightleftharpoons NDP\text{-}glucose + inorganic\ pyrophosphate\ (PP_i)$$

As we will see (§5.22), the pyrophosphorylase enzymes are considered to act as key sites in the regulation of polysaccharide synthesis.

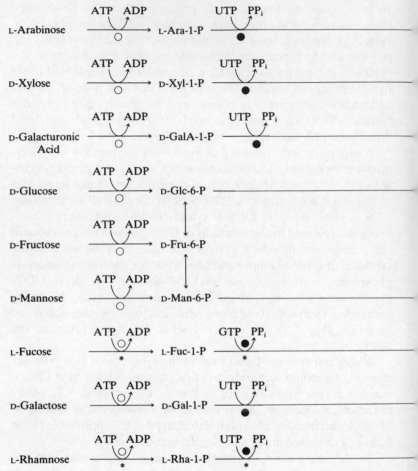

Fig. 5.2 Conversion of free monosaccharides to nucleotide sugars.
Ara, arabinose; Fru, fructose; Fuc, fucose; Gal, galactose; GalA, galacturoni◆
Glc, glucose; GlcA, glucuronic acid; GTP, guanosine triphosphate; Man, ma◆
Rha, rhammose; Xyl, xylose.

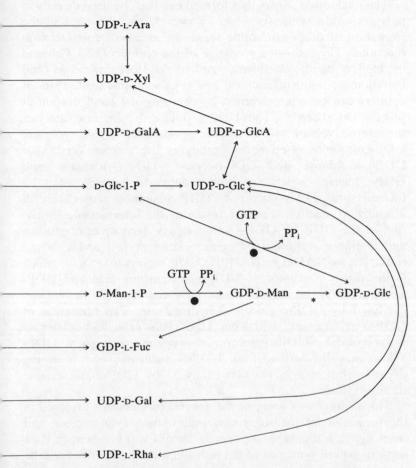

, preliminary evidence only available; ○, kinases; ●, pyrophosphorylases.

The nucleotide sugars thus formed can then be used directly in polysaccharide synthesis. Some, however, may be used in the formation of other nucleotide sugars by means of epimerization reactions. The following are some of the epimers (§2.1.1) found in higher plants: D-glucose and D-galactose; D-xylose and L-arabinose; D-glucuronic acid and D-galacturonic acid. Pairs of epimers can be interconverted by changing the configuration at just one chiral carbon. Thus UDP-D-glucose-4-epimerase catalyses the interconversion of UDP-D-glucose and UDP-D-galactose, and UDP-L-arabinose-4-epimerase catalyses the interconversion of UDP-L-arabinose and UDP-D-xylose. UDP-L-rhamnose and GDP-L-fucose, which are both 6-deoxyaldohexoses, may be formed from UDP-D-glucose and GDP-D-mannose respectively, in a multistep reaction sequence involving the intermediate formation of the UDP- or GDP-4-keto-6-deoxy derivatives of glucose and mannose, followed by epimerization at C-3 and C-5 and reduction by NADH or NADPH. UDP-D-glucuronic acid, which is the direct precursor of UDP-D-galacturonic acid and UDP-D-xylose, may be formed from UDP-D-glucose in a reaction catalysed by UDP-D-glucose dehydrogenase. The formation of UDP-D-galacturonic acid from UDP-D-glucuronate-4-epimerase is catalysed by UDP-D-glucuronate-4-epimerase. Finally, UDP-xylose may be derived from UDP-D-glucuronic acid following decarboxylation in a reaction catalysed by UDP-D-glucuronate decarboxylase.

This summarizes some of the general mechanisms involved in the formation of the sugar nucleotides, both from sucrose and from the free sugars. More specific details will be given in later sections where synthesis of the individual polysaccharides will be discussed.

5.2 Starch biosynthesis

Starch is the major reserve polysaccharide of green plants and is present in most types of tissue. Probably the most popular system used for studies on starch biosynthesis is that of the developing cereal endosperm. Experimentally the system has its advantages: firstly, the seeds mature over a relatively long period, enabling convenience of sampling and assay; secondly, a grain, seed or endosperm is a well-defined unit of fairly uniform size and hence results can be expressed on a unit basis; thirdly, many cereal cultivars or mutants exist which vary markedly in starch composition thus expanding the possibilities for biochemical and genetic investigations. Starch synthesis has also been studied in chloroplasts. While the mechanisms of synthesis may be similar in both amyloplasts and chloroplasts, the environmental conditions are very different. One major difference is that in chloroplasts starch turnover is rapid whereas in amyloplasts starch biosynthesis predominates.

5.2.1 Physiology of starch synthesis and accumulation

In cereal plants carbon fixed during photosynthesis in the stem, upper leaves and green parts moves to the developing seed where most of it is incorporated into starch within endosperm amyloplasts. The starch granules initially formed grow steadily in size within the surrounding double membrane, reaching a maximum average diameter in wheat of around 20–30 μm. When the seed attains maximum length there is a secondary formation of small starch granules. These are spherical, with a surrounding double

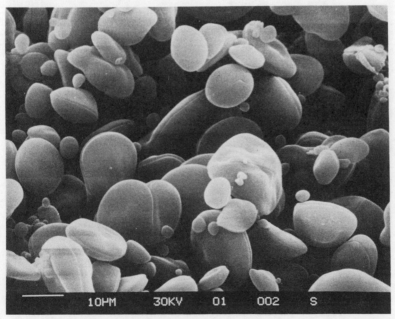

Fig. 5.3 Scanning electron micrograph of starch granules from immature wheat endosperm. Small granules are spherical, large granules have a characteristic lenticular shape with a peripheral groove.

membrane and have a maximum diameter of 10 μm. Their origins are unknown but it seems possible that they are formed by the blebbing off of peripheral regions of the large amyloplasts. In wheat, the large granules and those which are going to develop into large granules have a characteristic lenticular shape with a peripheral groove (Fig. 5.3). In electron micrographs of amyloplasts a tubular membranous complex can be seen at each end of the developing starch granule and within the outer membrane (Fig. 5.4). It may be that this is located in the groove surrounding the starch granule where it might act as the site of action of enzymes and cofactors involved in starch biosynthesis. Many plants other than the cereals are active in the synthesis of reserve starch. These include the legumes, e.g. peas and beans, the tubers,

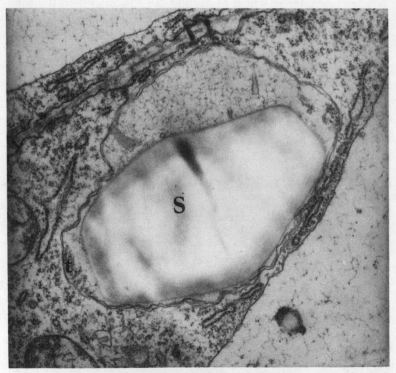

Fig. 5.4 Electron micrograph of amyloplast from an outermost starchy endosperm cell of a 19-day old caryopsis of barley cv. Midas. Tubuli **t** are present inside the amyloplast membrane at either end of the large starch granule S. (Reproduced by permission of Dr M. P. Cochrane.)

e.g. potatoes, yams and cassavas, and some tropical fruits, e.g. plantains, and mangoes. There seems to be little accumulation of starch in temperate fruits with the exception of apples where, in the cultivar Worcester Pearmain, maximum levels may approach 35 per cent (dry weight basis).

The variation in size, shape and complexity of starch granules is enormous and they are often used as aids in taxonomic identification. Those of the garden pea seed grow only to around 10 μm in diameter whereas those of potato may be as large as 100 μm in diameter. The characteristic morphological features of starch granules are not found in chloroplasts and are presumably a consequence not only of genetic influence but also of a relatively long period of starch synthesis uninterrupted by starch degradation.

In leaf chloroplasts, starch is synthesized during the day and is subsequently degraded at night or during periods when assimilate demand exceeds current photosynthetic production. The starch granules are very small and disc-shaped.

5.2.2 *Origin of substrates*

In tissues storing starch, sucrose is considered to be the primary substrate for starch synthesis (§3.6). The principal products of sucrose metabolism are UDP- and ADP-glucose, fructose and some glucose. Since the preferred nucleotide donor for starch synthesis is considered to be ADP-glucose, the principal fate of the three remaining products is probably conversion to ADP-D-glucose. In chloroplasts, the starch synthase is solely specific for ADP-D-glucose. This is derived from glucose-1-phosphate in a reaction catalysed by ADP-glucose pyrophosphorylase. In turn glucose-1-phosphate may be formed from fructose-6-phosphate, an intermediate of the photosynthetic carbon reduction cycle, via glucose-6-phosphate in reactions catalysed by phosphohexoisomerase and phosphoglucomutase.

Until about 1960 starch phosphorylase was the only enzyme known to catalyse the synthesis of α-(1→4)-D-glucans:

$$\text{D-glucose-1-phosphate} + (\text{glucosyl})_n \rightleftharpoons P_i + (\text{glucosyl})_{n+1}$$

Although phosphorylase activity increases in storage tissue during the period of starch synthesis, and also is present in chloroplasts, it has been questioned whether phosphorylase is functional in starch synthesis. The main reason for discounting phosphorylase is the reported high concentrations of P_i in relation to those of glucose-1-phosphate in both leaves and storage tissue. This would normally be expected to favour phosphorolysis rather than synthesis. Furthermore, starch synthesis by phosphorylase requires a relatively high concentration of glucose-1-phosphate. Amounts are low or undetectable and thus both in chloroplasts and storage tissue phosphorylase is considered to have a role in starch degradation (§6.1.4).

In 1961 Leloir, de Fekete and Cardini showed that the synthesis of α-(1→4)-D-glucan could be catalysed by starch synthase:

$$\text{ADP(UDP)-glucose} + (\text{glucosyl})_n \longrightarrow \text{ADP(UDP)} + (\text{glucosyl})_{n+1}$$

The sugar nucleotide precursors are in turn derived either from sucrose synthase (§3.6) or from glucose-1-phosphate in the reaction catalysed by the pyrophosphorylase enzyme (§5.1). All the plant ADP-glucose pyrophosphorylases so far investigated are subject to allosteric regulation, although those of storage tissues appear to be rather less sensitive. In general they are activated by 3-phosphoglycerate and inhibited by P_i. These effects help to explain how starch synthesis may be regulated in chloroplasts. During photosynthesis the production of ATP in photophosphorylation (§1.4.2) results in a lowered P_i concentration within the chloroplast. At the same time 3-phosphoglycerate levels rise due to increased carbon dioxide fixation. As a consequence ADP-glucose pyrophosphorylase is activated and starch begins to accumulate. In the dark, the P_i concentration rises and 3-phosphoglycerate levels fall as carbon is used in respiration. Starch synthesis is, therefore, prevented.

In storage tissue such as cereal endosperm, mechanisms controlling the levels of effectors and inhibitors are less well understood. Both UDP-glucose and ADP-glucose pyrophosphorylases are present throughout the period of starch accumulation. If ADP-glucose is indeed a major precursor of starch then much of the UDP-glucose synthesized by sucrose synthase (§3.6) must be channelled through glucose-1-phosphate to ADP-glucose via a combination of both UDP-glucose pyrophosphorylase and ADP-glucose pyrophosphorylase (Fig. 5.5). The developing amyloplast, like the chloroplast, is bounded by a double membrane. If the permeability of the amyloplast inner membrane is similar to that of the chloroplast, then there may be restrictions on the uptake of the intermediates of sucrose metabolism. It is possible, therefore, that many of the early reactions involved in starch synthesis take place within the developing amyloplast. That is, hexoses derived from

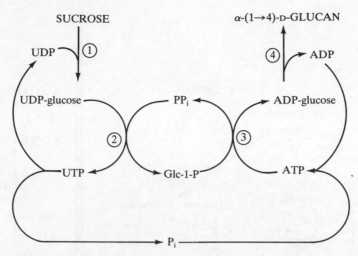

Fig. 5.5 Possible pathway for conversion of sucrose to α-D-(1→4)-glucan via UDP-glucose and ADP-glucose in developing cereal endosperm.
(1) UDP-dependent sucrose synthase; (2) UDP-glucose pyrophosphorylase; (3) ADP-glucose pyrophosphorylase; (4) starch synthase.
Catalytic amounts only of glucose-1-phosphate (Glc-1-P), nucleoside phosphates, pyrophosphate (PP_i) and inorganic phosphate (P_i) are required.

sucrose could be converted to dihydroxyacetone phosphate via glycolysis. Following uptake into the amyloplast this could be converted to ADP-glucose via gluconeogenesis and ADP-glucose pyrophosphorylase (Fig. 5.6).

5.2.3 Starch deposition

The starch of non-mutant reserve and chloroplast granules is a mixture of amylose and amylopectin (§2.3.1). All starches have a lower content of amylose than amylopectin and overall the amylose content is generally in the range 11–35 per cent. The amylose percentage varies almost as much among cultivars of a single species as among species. For example, the amylose percentage of maize starch ranges from 20–36 per cent, potato starch from 18–23 per cent and rice starch from 8–37 per cent.

The amylose content of most reserve starches increases with increasing age of the tissue examined. This has been observed in developing cereal grains, potato tubers and cassava roots. Thus

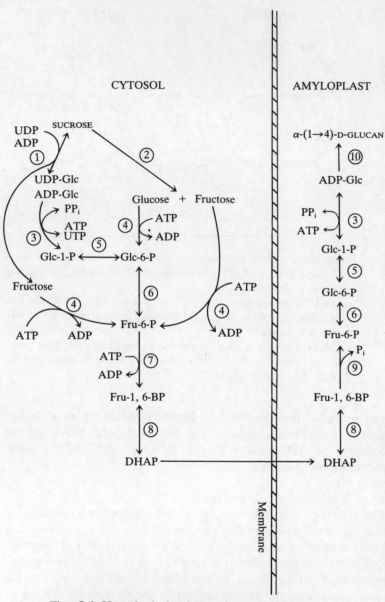

Fig. 5.6 Hypothetical scheme for conversion of sucrose to α-(1→4)-D-glucan assuming selective permeability of the amyloplast inner membrane.
(1) sucrose synthase; (2) invertase; (3) ADP-glucose and UDP-glucose pyrophosphorylases; (4) hexokinase; (5) phosphogluco-mutase; (6) phosphohexoisomerase; (7) phosphofructokinase;

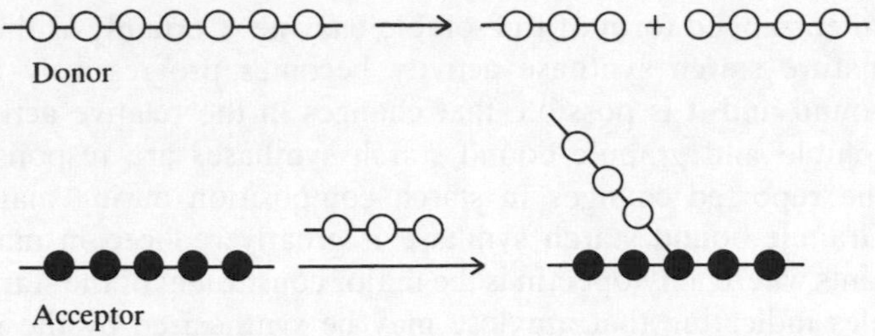

Fig. 5.7 Formation of α-(1→6)-glycosidic linkage by branching enzyme (Q-enzyme).
(1) Breaking of internal α-(1→4)-glycosidic linkage in donor α-(1→4)-D-glucan to form oligosaccharide chain.
(2) Formation of α-(1→6)-glycosidic linkage between acceptor glucan and oligosaccharide chain.

amylopectin synthesis must predominate at early stages of granule growth.

How the ratio of amylose to amylopectin is so closely controlled within a cultivar is still not understood but must presumably be a direct function of the enzymes involved. Starch synthase catalyses the stepwise addition of glucose residues to the non-reducing ends of maltodextrin primers with the formation of linear chains of α-(1→4)-linked D-glucose residues. Amylopectin is formed by the introduction of α-(1→6)-linkages into the straight chain molecules by the action of a branching enzyme (Q-enzyme) (Fig. 5.7). Since branching enzyme requires a continuous supply of α-(1→4)-D-glucan for activity it is likely that amylopectin synthesis is catalysed by the combined activities of both starch synthase and branching enzyme.

Starch synthases of storage tissues are often described as 'granule-bound' or 'soluble'. It is quite probable, however, that the 'soluble' activity is derived from stroma released by amyloplasts during extraction and that *in vivo* both types are localized within the amyloplast. It may be that the bound enzyme is merely

Caption to Fig. 5.6 (*cont.*)
(8) aldolase (simplified); (9) fructose-1,6-bisphosphatase; (10) starch synthase.
UDP-Glc, UDP-glucose; ADP-Glc, ADP-glucose; Glc-6-P, glucose-6-phosphate; Fru-6-P, fructose-6-phosphate; Fru-1, 6-BP, fructose-1, 6-bisphosphate; Glc-1-P, glucose-1-phosphate; DHAP, dihydroxyacetone phosphate; PP$_i$, pyrophosphate.

an entrapped form of the soluble enzyme. Certainly as the tissues mature starch synthase activity becomes progressively granule-bound and it is possible that changes in the relative activities of soluble and granule-bound starch synthases are responsible for the reported changes in starch composition during maturation. Granule-bound starch synthase is greatly reduced in maize mutants where amylopectin is the major constituent of the starch granules indicating that amylose may be synthesized by the granule-bound enzyme. Futhermore, amylopectin, which is the more soluble form of starch, predominates during the early stages of starch synthesis when starch synthase activity is mainly soluble. Hence it may be that amylopectin is synthesized by the soluble enzyme in association presumably with branching enzyme. The increase in amylose content as maturation proceeds may be explained by a progressive association between the granules and starch synthase.

Obviously, of course, branching enzyme activity influences the relative amounts of amylose and amylopectin formed. This enzyme catalyses the synthesis of amylopectin by cleaving a fragment from an α-D-glucan chain and transferring it to the C-6 position of an acceptor α-D-glucan (Fig. 5.7). The enzyme is difficult to assay, partly because most crude extracts are contaminated with amylases and partly because the reaction is not associated with a net synthesis of α-D-glucan. The simplest assay is to follow the decrease in absorbance of the amylose-iodine complex. However, this is unlikely to relate to any physiological situation since it measures the introduction of a few branches only into a linear substrate. A more satisfactory assay is that where branching enzyme is assayed by measuring its stimulation of unprimed synthesis of α-D-glucan from glucose-1-phosphate catalysed by phosphorylase a. The two enzymes are thought to act together, with phosphorylase catalysing elongation of the growing chain and branching enzyme introducing branch points. The synthesis of α-D-glucan is stimulated by the addition of branching enzyme since branching results in an increase in the number of non-reducing ends and hence an increase in the number of sites where elongation can proceed. Starch synthesis *in vivo* may have some relation to this process except that starch synthase replaces phosphorylase. Thus amylopectin synthesis probably proceeds by a combination of chain elongation and branching.

Starch synthase and branching enzyme are present in multiple forms in both leaves and reserve tissues. The role of these is imperfectly understood but it may be that they co-operate in the formation of different parts of the amylopectin molecule. How they are involved in the synthesis of a starch granule is unknown and indeed the complete formation of a starch granule *in vitro* has not yet been accomplished.

Little is known of the regulation of starch synthesis at the level of polymerization. Starch synthases require sugar nucleotides and α-D-glucan primers. The origin of the primers required for the initiation of starch synthesis is not known but it is possible that the cells contain endogenous maltodextrins which may act as primers. New primer molecules could be a result of amylase activity or even a result of unprimed synthesis by phosphorylase.

The starch synthases are unaffected by glycolytic intermediates but stimulated by univalent cations such as potassium. ADP is a competitive inhibitor with ADP-glucose. One of the multiple forms of branching enzyme, isolated using DEAE chromatography from maize endosperm, is coincident with starch synthase. This mixture will synthesize a branched polyglucan in the presence of citrate. Thus in the cell starch synthases may exist free or as a branching enzyme–starch synthase complex stabilized by citrate.

In sum, the mechanisms controlling the synthesis of starch are poorly understood and the precise nature of the genetic and biochemical factors which control the number, size, shape and composition of starch granules remains a mystery.

5.3 Biosynthesis of fructans and phytoglycogen

Almost half the fresh weight of Jerusalem artichoke tubers is present as β-$(2\rightarrow 1)$ linked fructans (inulin). Edelman and his colleagues have devised a scheme to show how they might be derived from sucrose. Initially it is considered that translocated sucrose is converted to a trisaccharide (isokestose) in the cytosol of tuber cells by a fructosyl transferase enzyme (Fig. 5.8). In a second reaction the terminal fructosyl group of the trisaccharide is transferred to a sucrose molecule by another fructosyl transferase enzyme on the tonoplast and the product, isokestose, enters the vacuole. Further transfers of terminal fructosyl groups from the trisaccharide molecules (Fig. 5.9) are thought to take place in the vacuole until chain termination takes place. It is envisaged that the sucrose released returns to the cytosol where it may be involved in the synthesis of new trisaccharide donors.

The β-$(2\rightarrow 6)$-linked fructans of grass have up to 50 β-D-fructofuranosyl residues and are the most abundant constituent

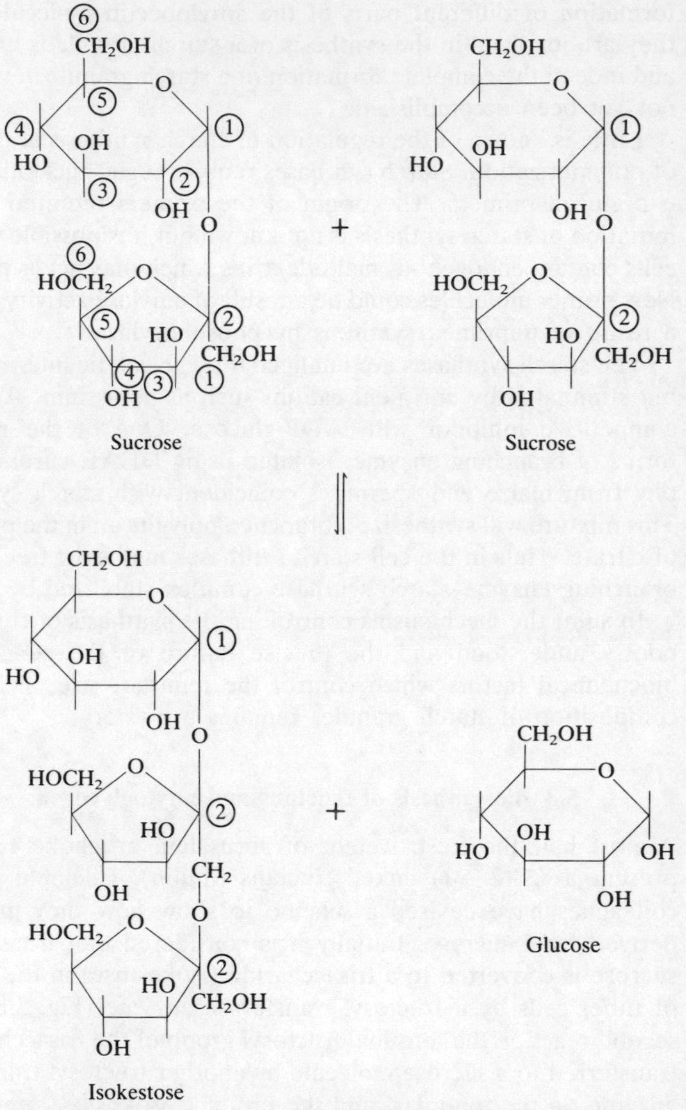

Fig. 5.8 Synthesis of isokestose from sucrose catalysed by sucrose–sucrose:1-fructosyl transferase.

of the water-soluble carbohydrate fraction of temperate grasses. The biochemical mechanisms concerned in their biosynthesis are poorly understood.

Two proposals have been put forward to explain the synthesis of phytoglycogen and starch in sweet corn endosperms. Firstly,

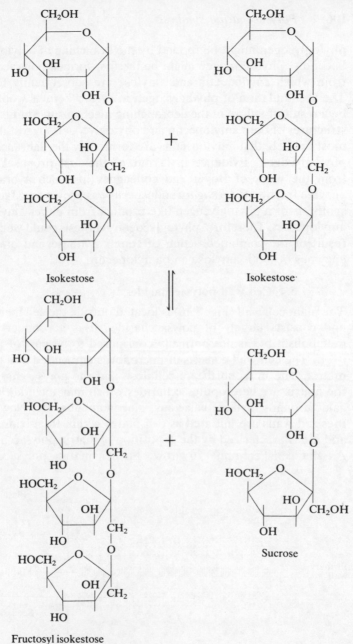

Isokestose   Isokestose

Fructosyl isokestose

⌐ Isokestose
└→ Sucrose

Higher homologues

Fig. 5.9 Synthesis of higher homologues of isokestose (inulin) from isokestose catalysed by β-$(2\rightarrow1)$-fructan: β-$(2\rightarrow1)$-fructan-1-fructofuranosyl transferase.

phytoglycogen might be formed by the branching of amylopectin. Secondly, phytoglycogen might be the first-formed polysaccharide from which amylopectin and amylose are subsequently formed. The accumulation of phytoglycogen in *sugary* kernels would then be a result of failure in the debranching mechanism. Studies of the structures of both amylopectin and phytoglycogen suggest that it is most unlikely that amylopectins are formed by the debranching of phytoglycogen. Evidence in favour of the first proposal comes from the work of Boyer and colleagues in which a branching enzyme fraction from *sugary* endosperm was shown to catalyse the synthesis of a phytoglycogen-like product from either amylose or amylopectin. Therefore, phytoglycogen synthesis could well be the result of the combined action of starch synthase and branching enzymes on both amylose and amylopectin.

5.4 Cell wall polysaccharides

The plant cell wall (Fig. 5.10) is located outside the cell membrane and consists largely of polysaccharide. It is a product of cell metabolism but is not normally considered to be part of the cell itself. The cell wall consists of microfibrils embedded in a gel-like matrix. The microfibrils are cellulose and the polysaccharides of the matrix are heteropolysaccharides which may include rhamnogalacturonans, xylans, galactans, glucomannans, etc. Newly synthesized walls are initiated as cell plates within the dividing cells and are characterized by the deposition of matrix polysaccharides. As the cells continue to grow, further matrix polysaccharide

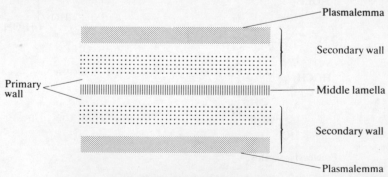

Fig. 5.10 Schematic representation of two adjacent cell walls. The secondary wall often consists of three layers. Thus the total cell wall may contain five layers, the middle lamella, the primary wall and a three-layered secondary wall.

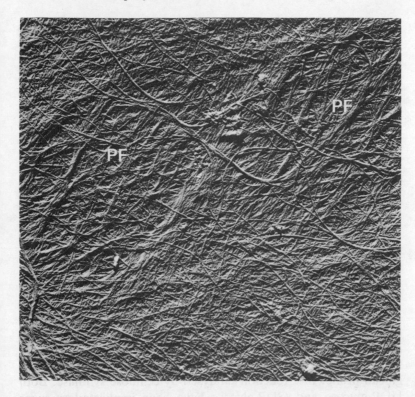

Fig. 5.11 Electron micrograph of the primary wall of a paren-chyma cell from wheat (*Triticum vulgare*) coleoptile, 10 mm from the tip (× 18,800). The microfibrils are in the form of a loose mat but with a predominantly transverse orientation, except in the lower left which represents an older part of the wall. Here the microfibrils are arranged in parallel and have more longitudinal orientation. Two pit fields (PF) are visible within which are localized numbers of plasmodesmata. Provided by Dr R. D. Preston, University of Leeds.

is laid down, together with microfibrils, thus forming the primary cell wall (Fig. 5.11). The adjacent cell walls are separated from each other by a layer between them called the middle lamella. It is likely that pectin is a major component of this layer. Further growth of the cell wall results in the formation of a secondary wall layer which, since it too is a product of cell metabolism, is located betwcen the cell membrane and the prim-ary wall. This is formed by cells that eventually form the harder, more woody portions of the plant. The secondary wall layer is often much thicker than the primary wall and has a characteristic polysaccharide composition and morphology. It has a higher proportion of microfibrils (cellulose) and a lower proportion of matrix material than the primary wall. It is composed of a succession of compact layers, in each of which the cellulose microfibrils lie parallel to each other. The fibrils of adjacent layers are generally oriented at different angles, an arrangement which is thought to confer strength to the cell wall.

Secondary cell walls may also contain the aromatic polymer lignin which gives rigidity to the cell walls and may be involved in the protection of cells against attack by pathogenic organisms. Characteristically lignified cells are those found in xylem where, apart from conferring rigidity, the lignin has a waterproofing effect on the conducting tissues by reducing the permeability of the cell walls.

5.4.1 Cellulose biosynthesis

Relatively little is known of the mechanism of cellulose biosynthesis in higher plants. The biosynthetic reaction is thought to involve the successive addition of glucosyl units from a sugar nucleotide donor to the non-reducing end of a β-(1→4)-linked glucan primer in a reaction catalysed by cellulose synthase. Both UDP-glucose and GDP-glucose have been implicated as sugar donors. The experimental results are conflicting, no doubt partly because the type of linkage formed seems to depend on the reaction conditions. Thus unless the reaction product is adequately characterized and shown to be a growing β-(1→4)-linked glucan polymer, it is difficult to identify specific donors, or indeed to investigate the mechanism of the reaction. Ultrastructural studies suggest (see Willison, 1981) that the cellulose microfibrils may be derived from an extracellular membrane-linked particulate complex. It may be that sugar nucleotides from the cell cytoplasm cross the plasmalemma where they are incorporated into the growing β-(1→4)-glucan chain. Alternatively, a polymeric precursor of cellulose, synthesized within the cell possibly in the Golgi apparatus, may pass by some means through the plasmalemma and on the outside become associated with other β-(1→4)-glucan polymers to form the microfibrils. It is not clear what triggers chain initiation and termination. While there is evidence that lipid-linked intermediates function in the transfer of monosaccharides between nucleotide sugars and cell wall polysaccharides in bacteria and fungi, it is still not entirely clear whether a similar system operates during cellulose synthesis in green plants.

Hopp and co-workers have outlined a cyclic scheme (Fig. 5.12) similar to that postulated for bacteria and based on their work with the green alga *Prototheca zopfii*, which suggests that a series of lipid-linked oligosaccharides may be involved in the synthesis of

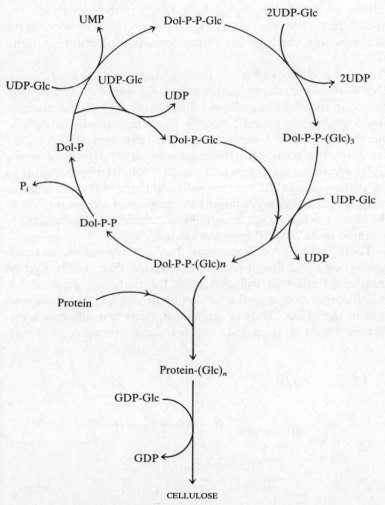

CELLULOSE

Fig. 5.12 Proposed scheme for the reactions leading to the formation of glycoproteins and cellulose (Hopp *et al.*, 1978). Dol, dolichyl.

cellulose. The lipid has some of the properties of dolichol, a term used to describe the group of polyprenols which have an α-saturated isoprene unit (Fig. 5.13). In this scheme glucose is transferred from UDP-glucose to dolichyl phosphate with the formation of a glucosyl-pyrophosphoryl-polyprenol. Subsequent reactions result in the formation of a β-$(1 \rightarrow 4)$-glucan derivative of dolichyl pyrophosphate. It is then postulated that the oligosaccharide moiety is transferred to an acceptor protein with the release of dolichyl pyrophosphate which is then recycled. The role of the GDP-glucose is seen to be that of a glucose donor in the final reaction which results in the formation of cellulose itself.

5.4.2 Biosynthesis of heteroglycans (see also §2.3.2)

The available evidence suggests that the enzyme systems concerned in the synthesis of non-cellulosic cell wall polysaccharides are located within the cell, probably in association with subcellular membranes. Several mechanisms have been suggested for their synthesis and transport. These include, firstly, synthesis in the Golgi apparatus, secretion into vesicles, followed by transport to the plasma membrane and, secondly, synthesis in the endoplasmic reticulum followed by transport to the plasma membrane. As in the case of cellulose synthesis the sugar nucleotide precursors are assumed to be derived from the cytosol.

These molecules contain more than one type of monosaccharide subunit and thus it has been suggested that specific glycosyl transferase enzymes will determine the particular monosaccharide incorporated as well as its anomeric configuration and position in the chain. Thus in arabinogalactans two different transferases would be required, one for the synthesis of β-$(1 \rightarrow 3)$-

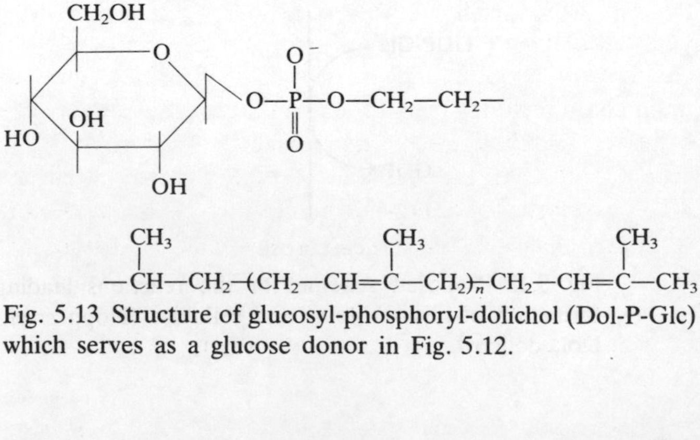

Fig. 5.13 Structure of glucosyl-phosphoryl-dolichol (Dol-P-Glc) which serves as a glucose donor in Fig. 5.12.

galactopyranose linkages and the other for the synthesis of β-$(1\rightarrow6)$-arabinofuranose–galactopyranose linkages.

Because of their complexity little is known of the mechanisms involved in the polymerization and assembly of heteroglycans. Ideally the reaction being investigated should demonstrate the synthesis of a high molecular weight product which is subsequently characterized and identified. In practice, however, the incorporation of only a few residues into an added primer is observed. That lipid intermediates may have a role in the biosynthesis of heteroglycans is suspected but little evidence is available to support this hypothesis.

The synthesis of pectic substances has probably received the greatest attention. The most active glycosyl donor for galacturonan synthesis is UDP-galacturonic acid. In pectin itself, the carboxyl groups of the galacturonic acid residues are methylated and this event appears to take place at the same time as, or very soon after, galacturonan polymerization. There is some evidence to suggest that the Golgi apparatus and its vesicles are concerned in pectin biosynthesis since pectic-type polysaccharides have been identified in these vesicles using pectinase degradation. Furthermore, the sugar residues associated with the Golgi apparatus are characteristically those of cell wall heteroglycans and include arabinose, galactose, glucose, xylose and uronic acids. That methylation follows polymerization and probably takes place in the Golgi-derived vesicles is suggested by analysis of pectic polysaccharides from both the Golgi apparatus and its secretory vesicles.

Most of the hemicellulose fraction of the cell wall of flowering plants consists of xylans. Like all heteroglycans their structure is complex. About half the xylosyl residues of the main chain are acetylated and short side chains contain 4-O-methyl-D-glucopyranosyluronic acid residues attached to C-2 of the xylosyl backbone residues by α-linkages. In monocotyledons the side chains also include L-arabinofuranose residues attached to the main chain residues by α-$(1\rightarrow3)$-linkages. Presumably these molecules are synthesized by the concerted action of a number of specific glycosyl transferases. While it seems clear that both UDP-D-xylose and UDP-L-arabinose act as sugar donors for the synthesis of arabinoxylan-type polysaccharides, little is known of the details of the enzymic reactions involved.

The cell wall itself consists of matrix and microfibrillar material as well as non-carbohydrate components such as protein, lignin and phenolic substances. Processes of self assembly and even active metabolism outside the plasmalemma may be involved in their synthesis and deposition.

5.4.3 β-Glucan synthesis

High rates of callose synthesis are observed in many plants following wounding or stress and the nucleotide sugar donor is probably UDP-glucose. As with many other complex macromolecules its synthesis and deposition are often studied using histochemical techniques. In this case cell wall material, which gives an intense bright yellow fluorescence with aniline blue, is generally referred to as 'callose' even though it cannot always be identified as a β-(1→3)-glucan. Using such methods it has been suggested that the β-(1→3)-glucan synthase responsible for callose synthesis is located at the plasma membrane. Callose is synthesized in the nucellar projection of immature cereal grains. This tissue lies on the route along which nutrients move from the vascular system of the parent plant to the developing endosperm. Speculation surrounds its possible function but it may be that it acts to regulate the uptake of nutrients and hormones into the developing seed.

Linear β-(1 → 3)(1 → 4)-D-glucans are synthesized during endosperm cell wall formation in cereals (§2.3.1) Since such β-glucans are notoriously difficult to characterize, little is known of the biochemical mechanisms involved. Interest in cell wall synthesis in barley endosperm stems from the fact that excessive release but incomplete hydrolysis of β-glucan during malting can result in slow filtration and lead to haze formation in high-gravity beers.

5.5 Biosynthesis of complex carbohydrates

5.5.1 Glycoproteins

The control of plant cell extension is thought to be mediated by processes which regulate the cross-linking of the cellulose network. It seems possible that the hydroxyproline-rich cell wall glycoprotein, extensin, is involved in this mechanism either by binding to other cell wall constituents such as polysaccharides, phenolics or lignin, or even by intramolecular interactions. It may be that the association of the peptide helix (§2.4) with the β-linked oligosaccharide gives rise to a collagen-like molecule, thus conferring flexibility and strength to the cell wall.

The formation of glycoproteins obviously involves the concerted action of both protein- and oligosaccharide-synthesizing systems. Hydroxyproline cannot be incorporated directly into protein as no base sequence exists to code for it. Thus proline residues are first incorporated into the peptide precursor and the hydroxyproline-rich peptide is then formed by post-translational hydroxylation of the proline residues. It is envisaged that synthesis of the polypeptide takes place in the rough endoplasmic reticulum. The mechanism whereby the newly synthesized polypeptide is incorporated into cell wall glycoprotein is not clear. Certainly UDP-arabinose appears to be a precursor of the arabinoside tri- or tetrasaccharide side chains and other evidence suggests that galactosylation of the serine residues takes place within the lumen of the endoplasmic reticulum.

The arabinogalactan proteins (AGPs) are referred to as β-lectins because they bind to β-glycosyl residues. Their biological role is obscure but they may be involved in cell-wall interactions. Like extensin, synthesis of the protein moiety probably involves post-translational hydroxylation of proline residues. The site of synthesis of the carbohydrate component, and whether or not it grows while attached to protein or is transferred as a unit, is unknown. It is not clear how the complete molecule is packaged and transported to its final location outside the plasma membrane.

5.5.2 Glycolipids

Glycolipids are characteristically found as components of plant cell membranes. For example, nearly half of the total lipid present in the chloroplast lamellar system is glycolipid, most of which is accounted for by mono- and digalactosyl diglycerides. Little is known of their biological function. The galactosyl donor is thought to be UDP-galactose and it has been suggested that the synthesis of monogalactosyl glycerol takes place by transfer of a galactose residue to diacyl glycerol:

diacyl glycerol + UDP-galactose $\longrightarrow$ monogalactosyldiglyceride + UDP

This product then serves as a precursor for the synthesis of digalactosyldiglyceride. The major site of synthesis is probably the chloroplast envelope.

Particulate enzyme preparations from a wide range of different plant tissues have been shown to catalyse the incorporation of glucose, derived from UDP-glucose, into steryl glucosides and acylated steryl glucosides:

$$\text{sterol} + \text{UDP-glucose} \xrightarrow{\text{transglucosylase}} \text{steryl glucoside} + \text{UDP}$$

Like the galactolipids, these molecules are found in plant cell membranes but their biological function is unknown.

Those glycolipids whose function is probably best understood are the lipid-linked saccharides for whom a role has been suggested in the synthesis of complex carbohydrates and cellulose. For example, the polyprenol dolichol has been implicated in the synthesis of cellulose (Fig. 5.12). A key intermediate is the β-(1 → 4)-linked glucan derivative of dolichyl pyrophosphate. It has also been suggested that polyprenol-linked monosaccharide intermediates may be involved in sugar transport across membranes, possibly as carriers of sugars for cell wall synthesis and protein glycosylation.

References

Bonner, J. and Varner, J. E (1976) *Plant Biochemistry*. Academic Press: New York.

Boyer, C. D., Damewood, P. A and Simpson, E. K. G. (1981) The possible relationship of starch and phytoglycogen in sweet corn, *Stärke* 33, 125–30.

Duffus, C. M. and Cochrane, M. P. (1982) Carbohydrate metabolism during cereal grain development, in *The Physiology and Biochemistry of Seed Development, Dormancy and Germination* (A. A. Khan, ed.). Elsevier/North Holland Biomedical Press: Amsterdam.

Edelman, J. and Jefford, T. G. (1968) The mechanism of fructosan metabolism in higher plants as exemplified in *Helianthus tuberosus*, *New Phytologist* 67, 517–31.

Franz, G. and Heiniger, U. (1981) Biosynthesis and metabolism of cellulose and noncellulosic cell wall glucans, in *Encyclopedia of Plant Physiology* (*Plant Carbohydrates II*), Vol. 13B (W. Tanner and F. A. Loewus, eds.). Springer-Verlag: Berlin.

Hopp, H. E., Romero, P. A., Daleo, G. R. and Pont Lezcia, R. (1978) Synthesis of cellulose precursors. The involvement of lipid-linked sugars, *Eur. J. Biochem.* 84, 561–71.

Jenner, C. F. (1982) Storage of starch, in *Encyclopedia of Plant Physiology* (*Plant Carbohydrates I*), Vol. 13A (F. A. Loewus and W. Tanner, eds.). Springer-Verlag: Berlin.

Lamport, D. T. A. and Catt, J. W. (1981) Glycoproteins and enzymes of the cell wall, in *Encyclopedia of Plant Physiology* (*Plant Carbohydrates II*), Vol. 13B (W. Tanner and F. A. Loewus, eds.). Springer-Verlag: Berlin.

Leloir, L. F., de Fekete, M. A. R. and Cardini, C. E. (1961) Starch and oligosaccharide synthesis from uridinediphosphate glucose, *J. Biol. Chem.* **236**, 636–41.

Preiss, J. and Levi, C. (1980) Starch biosynthesis and degradation, in *The Biochemistry of Plants*, Vol. 3 (P. K. Stumpf and E. E. Conn, eds.). Academic Press: New York.

Willison, J. H. M. (1981) Secretion of cell wall material in higher plants, in *Encyclopedia of Plant Physiology* (*Plant Carbohydrates II*), Vol. 13B (W. Tanner and F. A. Loewus, eds.). Springer-Verlag: Berlin.

6

Polysaccharide degradation

6.1 Starch degradation

Starch degradation appears to involve three stages (Fig. 6.1). Firstly, starch granules are broken down to maltodextrins, probably by α-amylase. Secondly, the maltodextrins are converted to glucose and glucose-1-phosphate. Thirdly, the glucose and glucose-1-phosphate are metabolized or transported to cells that require them.

6.1.1 α-Amylase

α-Amylase is a calcium-dependent enzyme which has been found in nearly every plant which has been studied. It hydrolyses α-(1→4)-linkages in both amylose and amylopectin to give a mixture of maltose and low molecular weight oligosaccharides. The pH optima of plant α-amylases tend to be in the acidic range, e.g. in cereals between 4.75 and 6.0. The 'α' in the name of the enzyme refers to the fact that the products of hydrolysis retain the α-configuration for some time and only slowly undergo mutarotation.

Amylose hydrolysis by α-amylase initially produces maltodextrins. The maltodextrins are then slowly hydrolysed at a rate inversely proportional to their chain length. The final products depend upon the concentration of the enzyme. With low concentrations of enzyme, traces of glucose, maltose, maltotriose and maltodextrins of 6–8 glucosyl units are the final products. With high concentrations of the enzyme, the products are maltose (about 90 per cent), maltotriose and glucose.

α-Amylase hydrolyses both the outer and inner chains of amylopectin but its action is hindered at the α-(1→6)-branch

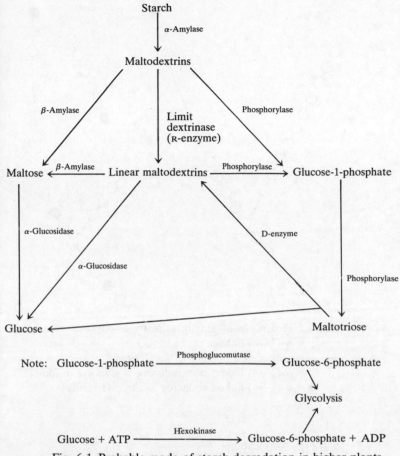

Fig. 6.1 Probable mode of starch degradation in higher plants.

points (Fig. 6.2). The products of hydrolysis are glucose, maltose, maltotriose and α-dextrins (branched oligosaccharides usually containing 5 to 10 glucosyl units).

Normally α-amylase will bind strongly to starch granules but this binding is inhibited by maltose and β-limit dextrins. Maltose has also been reported to inhibit degradation of starch granules. Thus, maltose may be an important regulator of α-amylase activity *in vivo* and there is evidence from studies of *Avena fatua* seeds that breakdown of maltose by maltase may be the key event in permitting starch breakdown to begin.

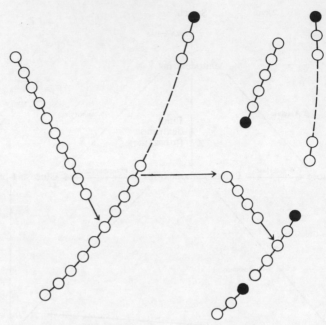

Fig. 6.2 Hydrolysis of amylopectin by α-amylase.
↓ = α-(1→6)-linkage
----- = unspecified portion of amylopectin
○ = α-(1→4)-linked non-reducing D-glucosyl residue
● = α-(1→4)-linked reducing D-glucosyl residue

6.1.2 β-Amylase

β-Amylase hydrolyses alternate α-(1→4)-linkages in starch-type polysaccharides releasing maltose from the non-reducing end(s) of the molecule (Fig. 6.3). Some amyloses are completely hydrolysed by β-amylase but others are not. Unlike α-amylase, it attacks only external chains of amylopectin and cannot bypass the α-(1→6)-branch points to attack the interior. Thus, the products of exhaustive hydrolysis of amylopectin by β-amylase are maltose and high molecular weight limit dextrins with two or three glucose residues external to the branch points. β-Amylase distribution in higher plants seems to be more restricted than that of α-amylase but it has been found in seeds, roots and leaves. The 'β' in the name of the enzyme refers to the mutarotation that occurs quite rapidly in maltose following hydrolysis so that the glycosidic linkage adopts the β-configuration.

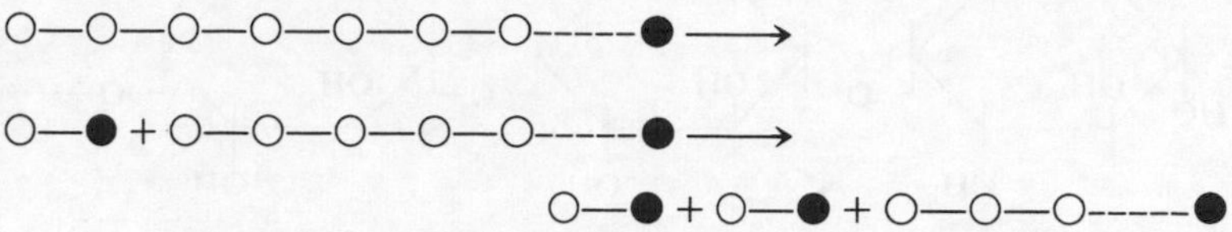

O—O—O—O—O—O—O-----● ⟶

O—● + O—O—O—O—O-----● ⟶

O—● + O—● + O—O—O-----●

Fig. 6.3 Stepwise action of β-amylase in hydrolysing chains of α-(1→4)-linked D-glucopyranose residues with the liberation of maltose.

O = α-(1→)-linked non-reducing D-glucosyl residue

● = α-(1→4)-linked reducing D-glucosyl residue

O—● = Maltose

----- = unspecified chain of α-(1→4)-linked D-glucosyl residues

β-Amylase is an enzyme that depends upon sulphydryl groups for its activity. When these groups are oxidized, activity is lost. This property is thought to allow the enzyme to be stored in ungerminated seeds in an inactive oxidized state ('latent' β-amylase). Activation of latent β-amylase may involve a protein disulphide reductase and possibly also proteolysis.

6.1.3 Phosphorylases

Phosphorylases in the presence of inorganic phosphate attack polysaccharides containing α-(1→4)-linked D-glucose residues releasing glucose-1-phosphate (Fig. 6.4). Phosphorylase will degrade amylose and the outer chains of amylopectin but it is probable that it can attack starch granules only after breakdown has been started by α-amylase.

Most of our knowledge of plant phosphorylases comes from studies of those isolated from potato and maize. Potato phosphorylase is a dimer containing pyridoxal phosphate and having a pH optimum at 6.5. Maize phosphorylase is also a pyridoxal-phosphate-containing dimer but with a pH optimum of 5.8. Neither of these phosphorylases appears to be regulated by phosphorylation and dephosphorylation like the mammalian liver phosphorylase. Both phosphorylases are capable of glucan synthesis given a primer of maltotriose or a higher glucan. The phosphorylases may be subject to allosteric inhibition by UDP-glucose.

6.1.4 α-Glucosidases

α-Glucosidases hydrolyse the α-(1→4)-linkages of dextrins from the non-reducing end, releasing glucose (Fig. 6.5). They are found

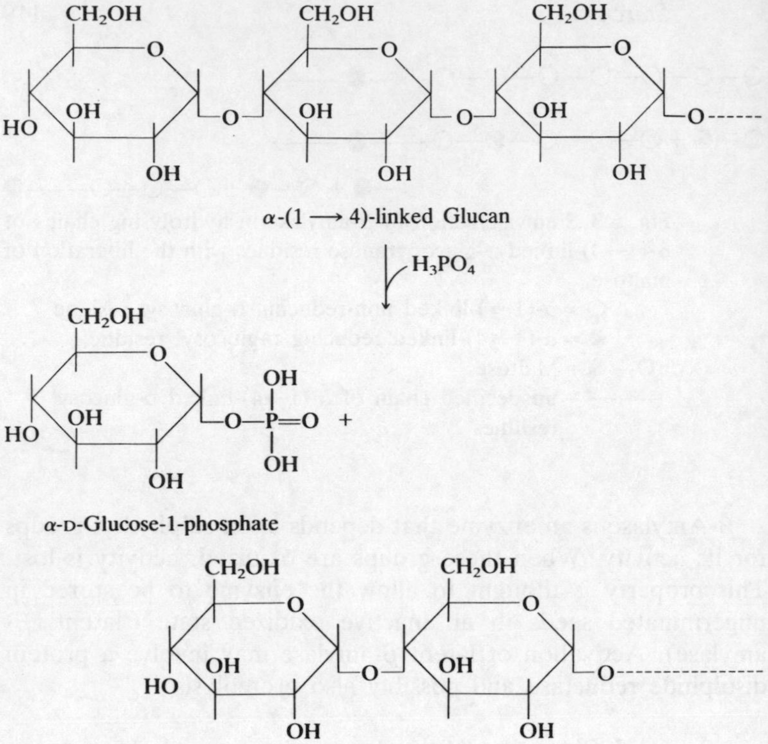

α-(1 $\longrightarrow$ 4)-linked Glucan

$\downarrow$ H_3PO_4

α-D-Glucose-1-phosphate

Fig. 6.4 Action of phosphorylases.

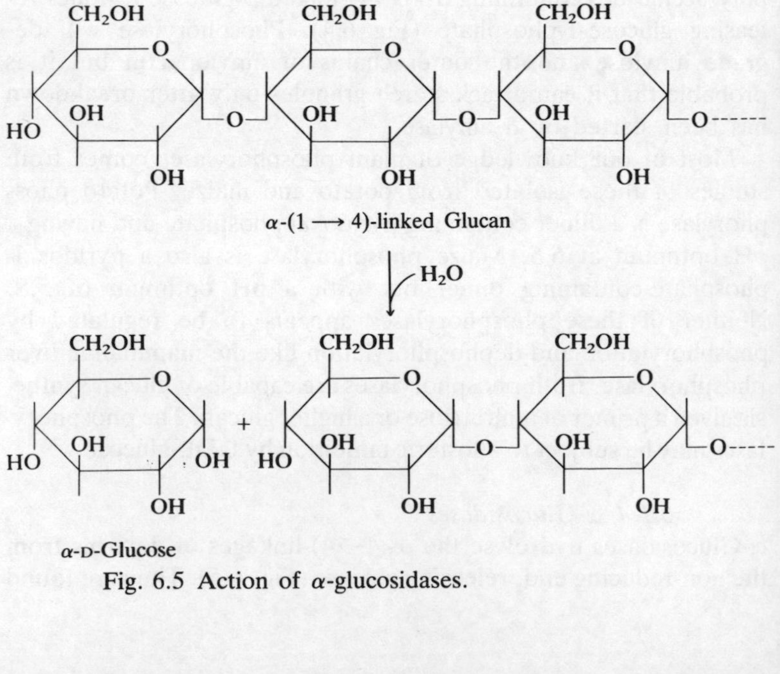

α-(1 $\longrightarrow$ 4)-linked Glucan

$\downarrow$ H_2O

α-D-Glucose

Fig. 6.5 Action of α-glucosidases.

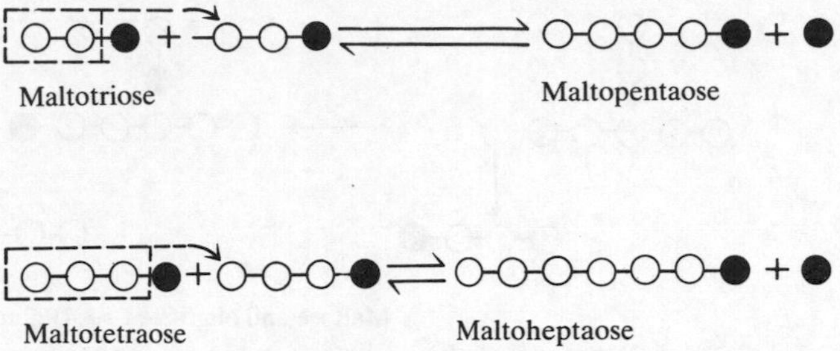

Fig. 6.6 Action of D-enzyme on maltotriose and maltotetraose. The transferred glucose residues are indicated by the dotted lines.

O = α-(1→4)-linked non-reducing D-glucosyl residue

● = α-(1→4)-linked reducing D-glucosyl residue

(from D. J. Manners, 1974. *In*:Essays in Biochemistry, Vol. 10 (P. N. Campbell and F. Dickens eds.) The Biochemical Society, London.

in most plants and can degrade maltotriose, maltotetraose, nigerose, dextrins, amylose, amylopectin and soluble starch. The pH optima are between 3 and 5. In some plants, the α-glucosidases occur as iso-enzymes.

6.1.5 D-enzyme

D-enzyme is a transglucosylase which catalyses the reversible condensation of α-(1→4)-glucans giving a redistribution of the glucosyl residues and releasing free glucose (Fig. 6.6). This enzyme can even use the outer chains of amylopectin as a substrate, transferring maltosyl or maltotriosyl units to an acceptor molecule which may be glucose or a glucan. The enzyme is found in a number of plants including potatoes, broad beans, carrots, tomatoes and maize.

The function of the enzyme in the living plant is uncertain but it may be either to produce primers for the synthesis of amylose or to help in starch degradation by producing from small limit dextrins larger molecules which can be readily attacked by phosphorylase.

6.1.6 Debranching enzymes

Debranching enzymes hydrolyse the α-(1→6)-D-glucosidic linkages in amylopectin and α-dextrins (Fig. 6.7). At one time a

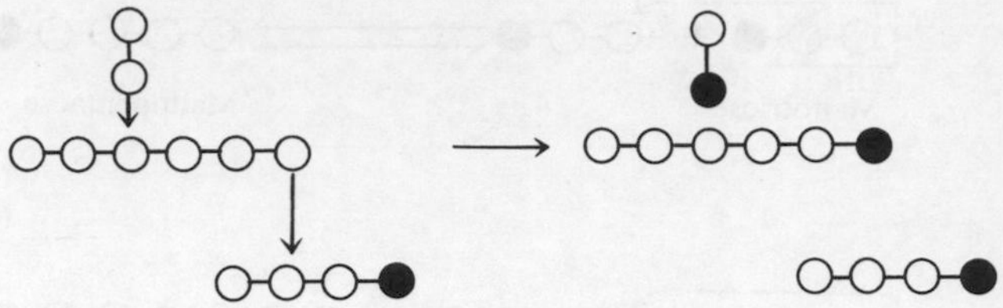

Maltose and oligo-α-(1 → 4)-glucosides

Fig. 6.7 Action of debranching enzymes
↓ = α-(1→6)-linkage
O = α-(1→4)-linked non-reducing D-glucosyl residue
● = α-(1→4)-linked reducing D-glucosyl residue
(From D. J. Manners. 1974. See caption for Figure 6.6 for details.)

distinction was made between limit dextrinases, which were supposed to be active only on α-limit dextrins, amylopectin, β-limit dextrins and pullulan, and R-enzymes which could also attack α-(1→6)-linkages in amylopectin. It is now clear that this distinction is invalid as dilution of R-enzyme solutions decreases their action on amylopectin to a point where it is virtually undetectable and the enzyme is thus indistinguishable from limit dextrinase. Because of this, some workers classify all plant debranching enzymes as pullulanases (§9.3.3). However, in this text the R-enzyme and limit dextrinase terminology will be retained wherever the distinction is still found commonly in the literature.

6.1.7 Starch degradation during germination and malting
Much of our knowledge of starch degradation comes from studies of seed germination and especially from studies on barley. Barley germination is the essential process in making malt, the raw material of brewing; the economic importance of the process has provided the main impetus for research in this area. Germination of barley is accompanied by increases in activity of α-amylase and β-amylase. β-Amylase occurs in barley in 'free' and 'latent' forms (see also 6.1.3). 'Free' β-amylase appears to be derived from the 'latent' form which is the same enzyme bound to the protein glutein. Conversion of 'latent' β-amylase to the 'free' form can be brought about *in vitro* by thiol reducing agents and it may be that *in vivo* conversion is a similar process catalysed by a disulphide reductase. Thus, it appears that β-amylase is present in ungerminated barley in the 'latent' inactive form and that the increase in

activity during germination is due to the conversion (activation) process which follows the release of gibberellins from the embryo or their exogenous application.

Unlike β-amylase, α-amylase is synthesized *de novo* during germination. This synthesis occurs in the aleurone layer of barley and is triggered by endogenous or exogenous gibberellin. Following synthesis, the α-amylase is secreted into the endosperm. In seeds other than barley, α-amylase synthesis may occur in the scutellum as has been reported for maize.

In addition to the amylases, other hydrolytic enzymes increase in activity during germination. These include R-enzyme, β-glucanases, pentosanases and maltase. The β-glucanases and pentosanases are important in relation to starch breakdown in that they break down endosperm cell walls which form a mechanical barrier preventing amylases from coming in contact with starch granules.

6.1.8 Starch degradation in leaves

Starch comprises about 1 per cent of the dry weight of leaves where it forms a temporary store of carbohydrate made by photosynthesis. At night the starch is converted back to sugars which are transported to non-photosynthetic tissues.

Since starch in most higher plant leaves is restricted to chloroplasts, it might be expected that starch-degrading enzymes would also be detectable in these organelles. This is true for α-amylase, phosphorylase and R-enzymes but not so far for β-amylase. β-Amylase appears to be located in the cytoplasm of leaf cells, along with the major portion of the activity of the other enzymes that have been studied.

Investigation of starch degradation in leaves shows that the major products are 3-phosphoglycerate, maltose, sometimes glucose, and small amounts of glucose-6-phosphate and ribose-5-phosphate. It is probable that phosphorylase initiates all the conversion of starch to sugar phosphates and that α- and/or β-amylases account for maltose and glucose production.

6.2 Degradation of other polysaccharides

6.2.1 Introduction

Although starch is the most common storage polysaccharide in plants, other polysaccharides can have a storage function. These include fructans in the Compositae and some grasses, galactomannans in the Leguminosae and xyloglucans in the seeds of several families. Enzymes exist for the degradation of all these polysaccharides but much work remains to be done on their characterization.

In addition to storage polysaccharides there are structural polysaccharides in the plant cell wall. The main cell wall polysaccharide is cellulose which is in the form of fibres embedded in a matrix of other polysaccharides such as xyloglucan, arabinoxylan, glucans, xylans, mannans, galactans and pectic substances (galacturonan, arabinan and galactan). Although cell wall polysaccharides are fairly stable, plants produce hydrolases which can modify them and break them down. This can be seen when end walls are degraded in the formation of xylem vessels and phloem sieve tubes or during leaf abscission and fruit ripening. A dramatic example of such hydrolase activity is the action of pollen tubes as they pass through the style, dissolving the wall in their path. It is even likely that all plant cell growth depends to some extent on hydrolase activity to permit loosening of the wall structure and the insertion of new material.

In this section, only a few of the enzymes involved in the degradation of non-starch polysaccharides will be discussed. The enzymes to be described have been selected only on the basis of availability of information and it should not be assumed that they are necessarily the most important enzymes.

6.2.2 Cellulases

Cellulases are enzymes which hydrolyse β-$(1\rightarrow4)$-glucans (Fig. 6.8). Their main function is probably to weaken cell walls to permit growth and differentiation, or abscission of flowers, seeds and leaves. It seems unlikely that they have any digestive role permitting cellulose to be used by plants as a carbon source.

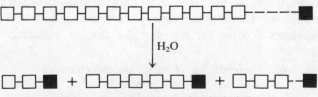

β-Glucans produced by random hydrolysis

Fig. 6.8 Action of cellulases
$\square$ = β-$(1\rightarrow4)$-linked non-reducing D-glucosyl residue
$\blacksquare$ = β-$(1\rightarrow4)$-linked reducing D-glucosyl residue

The pH optimum of cellulases is usually between 4.5 and 7.0. They preferentially attack interior linkages of cellulose in what appears to be a fairly random manner producing oligoglucosides. For complete conversion of cellulose to glucose, β-glucosidases ('cellobiases') must be present to degrade the oligoglucosides.

6.2.3 β-Glucanases other than cellulase
Apart from cellulase, endo-β-glucanases have been identified that can hydrolyse β-(1→3)-linkages and adjacent β-(1→3)- and β-(1→4)-linkages. It is thought that these enzymes are particularly important in the breakdown of the endosperm cell walls in germinating seeds. Initially the β-glucan is solubilized by an acidic carboxypeptidase known as β-glucan solubilase and then the endo-β-glucanases degrade the solubilized material to oligosaccharides. These, in turn are converted to glucose by β-glucosidase enzymes.

6.2.4 Fructan hydrolases
Fructan hydrolases attack only β-(2→1)-fructofuranoside linkages in straight chain oligosaccharides and polyfructosides of the inulin series (Fig. 6.9). Most studies have been carried out on the inulin-1-fructanohydrolase from Jerusalem artichoke tubers. This enzyme has a pH optimum between 5.0 and 5.5 and removes single fructose residues from the non-reducing chain ends of the substrate.

6.2.5 Other polysaccharide hydrolases
Various polysaccharide hydrolases other than those mentioned above have been identified in plant tissues. The enzymes found include β-glucosidases, α- and β-galactosidases, α-mannosidases, arabinosidases, *exo-* and *endo*-xylanases, and β-N-acetylhexosaminidase. All of these enzymes apart from the *endo*-xylanases remove terminal residues, generally but not always from low molecular weight substrates. Their pH optima are usually in the acidic range.

It will be clear to the reader that there must be many polysaccharide hydrolases in plant tissues which have not been mentioned. Their omission reflects the neglect which this area of study has suffered and it is to be hoped that the current interest in plants as renewable resources of chemical feedstocks may stimulate the research that is needed to permit a more complete understanding of these enzymes and their functions.

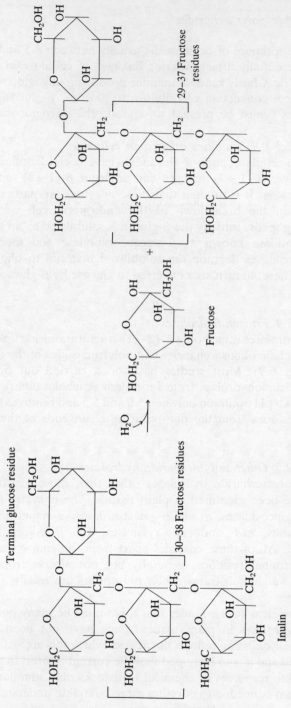

Fig. 6.9 Action of fructan hydrolases.

References

Aspinall, G. O. (1970) *Polysaccharides*. Pergamon Press.

Aspinall, G. O. (1972) Degradation of polysaccharides, in *Weissberger's Techniques of Organic Chemistry*, Vol. IV, Elucidation of Structures (2nd edn.) (K. W. Bentley and G. W. Kirby eds.). Wiley: New York.

Aspinall, G. O. (ed.) 1982 The Polysaccharides, Vol. 1, Academic Press.

Aspinall, G. O. and Stephen, A. M. (1976) Polysaccharide methodology and plant polysaccharides, in *Carbohydrates* (MTP International Review of Science, Organic Chemistry Series Two, Vol. 7) (Consultant ed. D. H. Hey F. R. S.; Volume ed. G. O. Aspinall). Butterworths.

Boyer, P. D. ed. (1972) *The Enzymes* (2nd edn.), Vol. V, Hydrolysis (Sulphate Esters, Carboxyl Esters, Glycosides), Hydration. Academic Press: New York.

Ginsburg, V. ed. (1972) *Methods in Enzymology*, Vol. XXVIII, Complex Carbohydrates, Part B (S. P. Colowick and N. O. Kaplan, series eds.). Academic Press: New York.

Ginsburg, V. and Robbins, P. (1981) *Biology of Carbohydrates*, Vol. I. Wiley: New York.

Hall, J. L., Flowers, T. J. and Roberts, R. M. (1982) *Plant Cell Structure and Metabolism* (2nd edn.). Longman.

Manners, D. J. (1974) The structure and metabolism of starch, in *Essays in Biochemistry*, Vol. 10 (P. N. Campbell and F. Dickens eds.). Academic Press.

Neufeld, E. F. and Ginsburg, V. (1966) *Methods in Enzymology*, Vol. III, Complex Carbohydrates (S. P. Colowick and N. O. Kaplan, series eds.). Academic Press: New York and London.

Preiss, J and Levi, C. (1979) Metabolism of starch in leaves, in *Encyclopedia of Plant Physiology New Series*, Vol. 6, Photosynthesis II (M. Gibbs and E. Latzko, eds.). Springer-Verlag: Berlin.

7

Secondary products

7.1 The definition of secondary products

The division of plant compounds into primary and secondary products is traditional. Secondary products were originally defined as those compounds which are not essential to the survival of the plant and which are not widely distributed in the plant kingdom. However, it is now clear that many compounds, long established as secondary products, are in fact performing vital functions as hormones, insect attractants, antifungal agents, etc. Further, improved analytical techniques have shown that many secondary products are ubiquitous in the plant kingdom. Thus, the original definition is no longer valid though the segregation of compounds into primary and secondary products persists. For the purposes of this book, the secondary products of carbohydrate metabolism to be discussed will be the cyclitols, glycosides, exudate gums and seaweed gums, though this is a purely arbitrary selection.

7.2 Cyclitols

Cyclitols are carbocyclic compounds with several hydroxyl groups. The most widely occurring cyclitols are inositols and quercitols. Inositols have a six-membered carbon ring with six hydroxyl groups. Quercitols also have a six-membered ring but with only five hydroxyl groups.

The most studied of the cyclitols is *myo*-inositol (= *meso*-inositol), a sugar alcohol found in all plants. It is synthesized from D-glucose-6-phosphate by way of *myo*-inositol-1-phosphate which is dephosphorylated by a specific phosphatase (Fig. 7.1). *Myo*-inositol is the precursor of all the other naturally occurring inositols as shown in the figure.

Inositols are converted to uronic acids. For example, D-glucuronic acid is formed from *myo*-inositol (Fig. 7.1). The UDP derivative of glucuronic acid may be further converted to UDP-galacturonic acid and hence to pectins or, alternatively, to certain pentoses or to the branched sugar, D-apiose (Fig. 7.2). It is thought that methylated inositols may be the precursors of the methylated sugars in plant cell walls.

Myo-inositol-1-phosphate is the compound from which phytic acid (*myo*-inositol hexaphosphate) is formed by phosphorylation, phosphate groups being derived from ATP. Phytic acid is an important storage form of phosphate in higher plants, especially in seeds.

Myo-inositol synthesized in chloroplasts takes part in the transport of sugar residues through the chloroplast membrane into the cytoplasm. *Myo*-inositol also forms esters with the plant growth regulator 3-indolylacetic acid (auxin). These esters may be involved in the modification of cell walls. Methyl ethers are formed readily from *myo*-inositol and these may be the precursors of methylated polysaccharides. *Myo*-inositol is also a precursor of phospho-inositides which are complex glycolipids. The complex galactinol (1-*O*-α-D-galacto-pyranosyl-*myo*-inositol) is formed by combination of *myo*-inositol with galactose. Galactinol transfers galactosyl residues to sucrose, raffinose and higher homologues of raffinose (Fig. 7.3). The reaction is reversible.

7.3 Glycosides

Glycosides are the compounds formed when sugars combine among themselves or react with non-carbohydrates with the formation of glycosidic linkages. However, the term tends to be used most frequently to cover the latter group. The non-sugar moiety is known as the aglycone or genin (Fig. 7.4). The most common glycosides are the *O*-glycosides (Fig. 7.4) where the sugar is linked through the oxygen atom to an alcohol, phenol or acid. The sugar can also be linked directly to a carbon atom (*C*-glycoside), to a nitrogen atom (*N*-glycoside), or to a sulphur atom (*S*-glycoside). Aglycones can be phenols, terpenoids, steroids or various nitrogen- and sulphur-containing compounds. D-Glucose is the most common sugar to be found in glycosides. It is the only sugar in the *S*-glycosides which are known as glucosinolates (Fig. 7.5). It is also the main sugar in cyanogenic glycosides (Fig. 7.6). D-Galactose, D-xylose, L-rhamnose and L-arabinose are

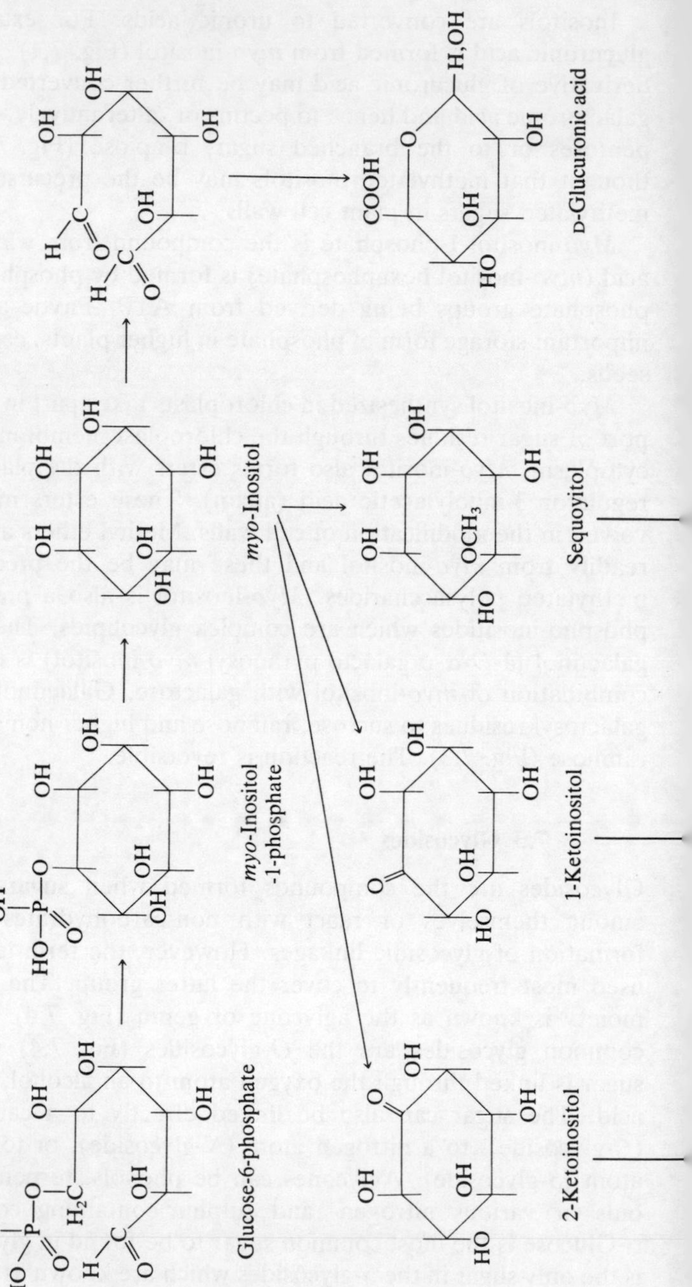

D-Glucuronic acid

myo-Inositol

Sequoyitol

myo-Inositol -1-phosphate

1-Ketoinositol

Glucose-6-phosphate

2-Ketoinositol

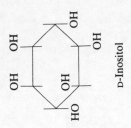

Fig. 7.1 Synthesis of inositols and their derivatives.

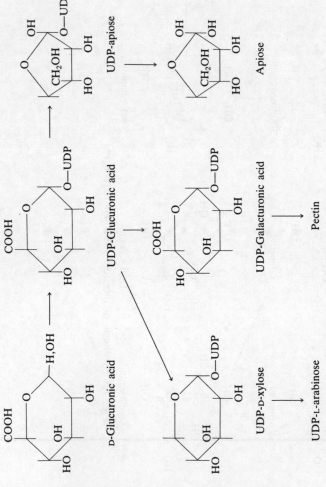

Fig. 7.2 Synthesis of derivatives of glucuronic acid.

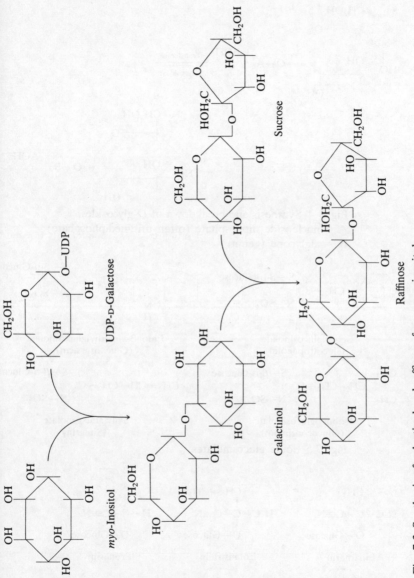

Fig. 7.3 Synthesis of galactinol and raffinose from *myo*-inositol.

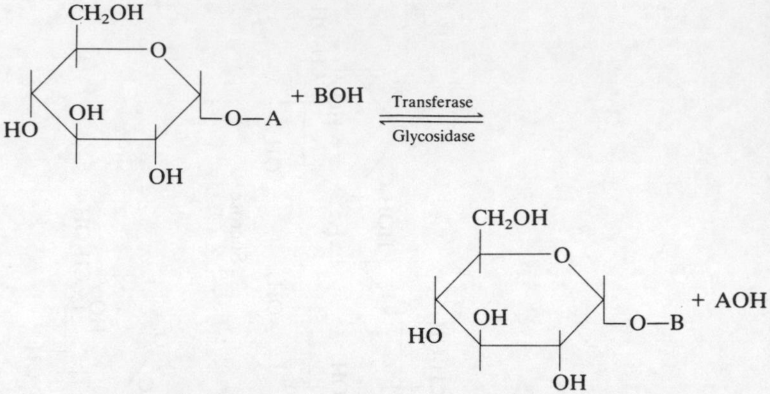

Fig. 7.4 Synthesis and breakdown of *O*-glycosides.
A = nucleoside diphosphate (often uridinediphosphate)
B = alglycone (genin)

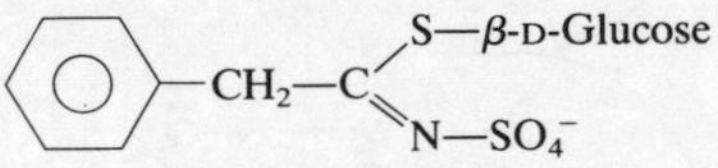

Benzylglucosinolate
(Glucotropaeolin)

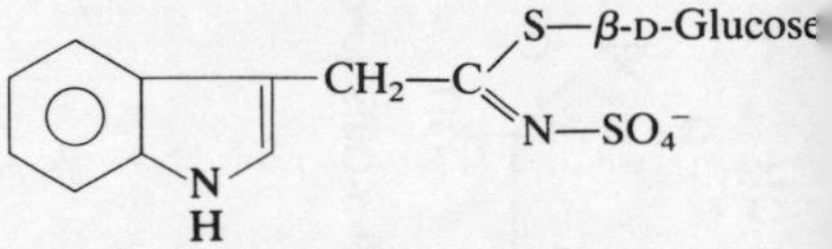

Indol-3-ylmethylglucosinolate
(Glucobrassicin)

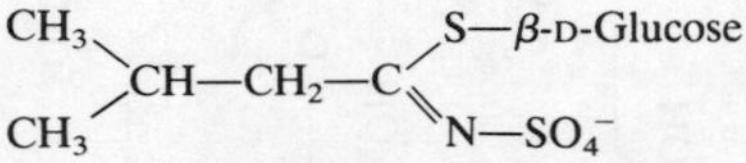

Isobutylglucosinolate
(Glucoconringiin)

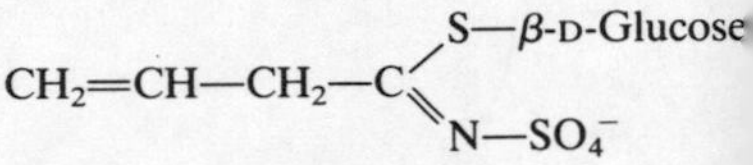

Allylglucosinolate
(Sinigrin)

Fig. 7.5 Some glucosinolates.

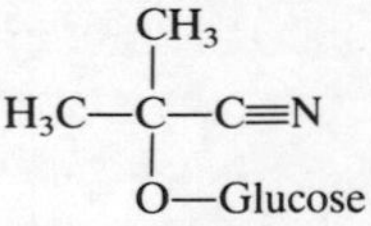

Linamarin

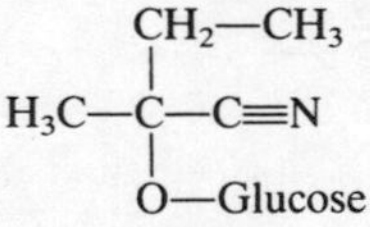

Lotaustralin

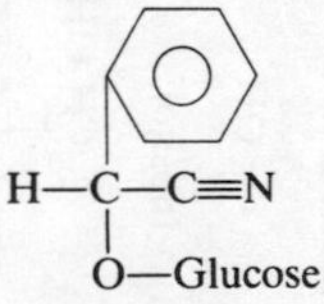

Prunasin

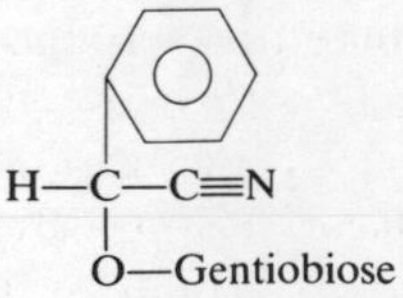

Amygdalin

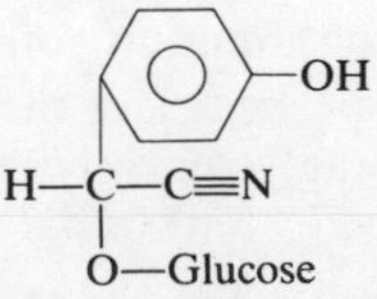

Dhurrin

Fig. 7.6 Some cyanogenic glycosides.

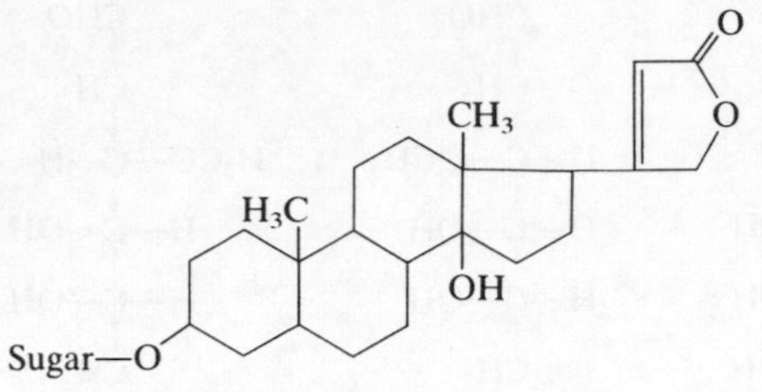

Cardenolide type

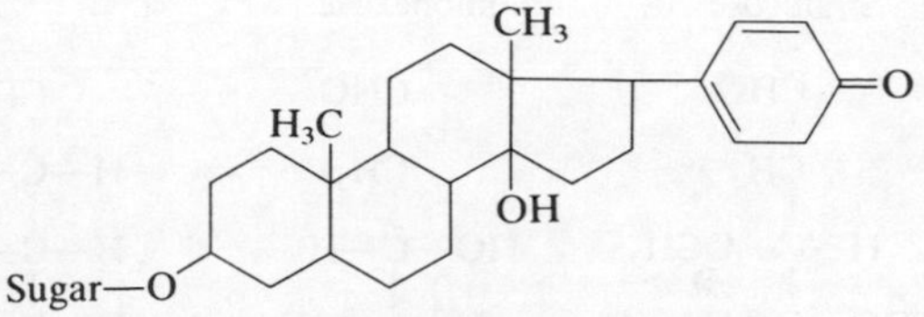

Bufadienolide type

Fig. 7.7 Cardiac glycosides.

other sugars commonly found in glycosides but D-fructose is quite rare. Some of the monosaccharides found in cardiac glycosides (Fig. 7.7) are quite unusual. These include 6-deoxy-D-glucose and 2-deoxy-D-arabinohexose and other 6-deoxy- and 2-deoxy-derivatives. Deoxymethylpentoses (2,6-dideoxy-sugar methyl ethers) are common among cardiac glycosides but are not found in other types of glycoside. Some examples of deoxymethylpentoses (cymarose, oleandrose, sarmentose and diginose) are shown in Fig. 7.8. D-Diginose is found in African *Strophanthus* species while the L-isomer is found in Asian species. D-Fucose occurs in cardiac glycosides only but L-fucose is ubiquitous.

Diglycosides are somewhat rare though disaccharides are found in association with aglycones. For instance, gentiobiose occurs in flavonols and anthocyanins in *Primula sinensis* and in amygdalin in members of the Rosaceae. Another disaccharide, vicianose, has been found in violutoside, a salicylic acid ester from *Viola cornuta*, and in vicianin, a cyanogenic glycoside from *Vicia angustifolia*.

Oligoglycosides are quite common, often linked to terpenoid aglycones as in the saponins. The sugars are usually attached to the 3-hydroxyl group of the aglycone. However, in the saponin gypsoside A (Fig. 7.9) from *Gypsophila pacifica*, the branched chain oligosaccharides are attached to two hydroxyl groups of the terpenoid aglycone. The cardiac glycosides also may contain oligosaccharides.

```
     CHO              CHO              CHO              CHO
      |                |                |                |
 H—C—OH             CH2              CH2              CH2
      |                |                |                |
HO—C—H           HO—C—H          H—C—OCH3       H3CO—C—H
      |                |                |                |
 H—C—OH           H—C—OH           H—C—OH           H—C—OH
      |                |                |                |
 H—C—OH           H—C—OH           H—C—OH           H—C—OH
      |                |                |                |
     CH3             CH2OH             CH3              CH3

 6-Deoxy-        2-Deoxy-D-        D-Cymarose        D-Oleandrose
 D-glucose       arabinohexose
```

```
     CHO              CHO              CHO              CHO
      |                |                |                |
     CH2              CH2           H—C—OH             CH2
      |                |                |                |
 H—C—OCH3         HO—C—H           H—C—OH           H—C—OCH3
      |                |                |                |
HO—C—H            H—C—OH           H—C—OH           HO—C—
      |                |                |                |
HO—C—H            H—C—OH           H—C—OH           H—C—OH
      |                |                |                |
     CH3             CH2OH             CH3              CH3

 L-Oleandrose     2-Deoxy-         6-Deoxy-        D-Sarmentose
                  D-glucose        D-allose
```

```
     CHO              CHO              CHO              CHO
      |                |                |                |
     CH2              CH2           H—C—OH           H—C—OH
      |                |                |                |
H3CO—C—H          H—C—OCH3         H—C—OH           H—C—OH
      |                |                |                |
HO—C—H            H—C—OH           HO—C—H           H—C—OH
      |                |                |                |
 H—C—OH           HO—C—H           H—C—OH           HO—C—H
      |                |                |                |
     CH3              CH3              CH3              CH3

 D-Diginose       L-Diginose       6-Deoxy-         6-Deoxy-
                                   D-gulose         L-talose
```

```
     CHO              CHO              CHO
      |                |                |
 H—C—OH           HO—C—H           H—C—OH
      |                |                |
HO—C—H            H—C—OH           H3CO—C—H
      |                |                |
HO—C—H            H—C—OH           H—C—OH
      |                |                |
 H—C—OH           HO—C—            H—C—OH
      |                |                |
     CH3              CH3              CH3

 D-Fucose         L-Fucose         D-Thevetose
```

Fig. 7.8 Some unusual monosaccharides found in cardiac glyco-sides.

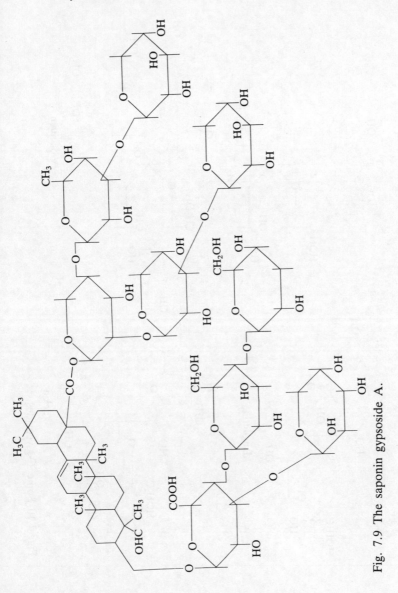

Fig. 7.9 The saponin gypsoside A.

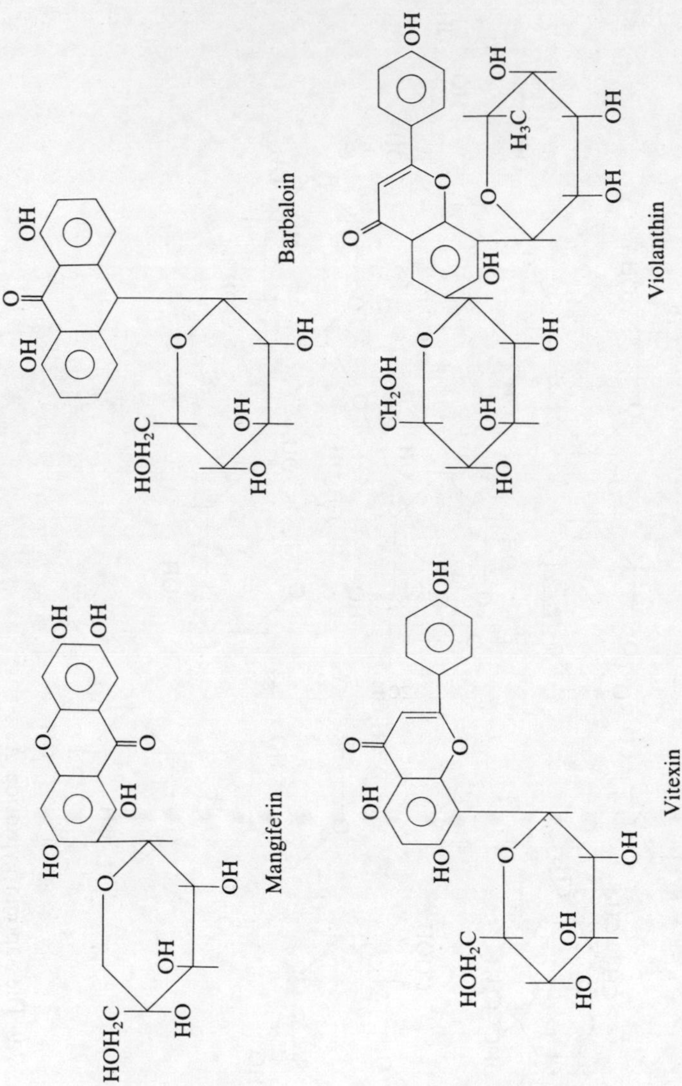

Fig. 7.10 Some C-glycosides.

C-glycosides are not as common as *O*-glycosides. They include mangiferin, first found in the roots of *Mangifera indica*; barbaloin, from *Aloe* species; vitexin, originally isolated from *Vitex lucens*; and violanthin from *Viola tricolor* (Fig. 7.10).

N-glycosides are most obviously represented by the D-ribose and D-deoxyribose derivatives of purines and pyrimidines, that is to say, the nucleosides, nucleotides and nucleic acids.

A number of glycosides are toxic to animals, usually owing to an effect of the aglycone. All cardiac glycosides and saponins can damage cell membranes, upsetting the ionic balance, and this can ultimately lead to heart stoppage and death. However, such effects usually only follow injection into the blood stream. In the digestive tract the sugars are hydrolysed from the aglycones which usually cannot pass readily through the gut wall.

Cyanogenic glycosides can release hydrogen cyanide following enzymic hydrolysis and this is the basis of their toxicity to animals. Glucosinolates also yield toxic products – cyanides, thiocyanates and isothiocyanates (mustard oils) – after hydrolysis by specific enzymes (Fig. 7.11). Only one of the enzymes, myrosinase or thioglucoside glucohydrolase (responsible for isothiocyanate formation), has been characterized. The isothiocyanates are particularly noted for their goitrogenic effects.

Ranunculin from buttercups can be enzymically converted to protoanemonin (Fig. 7.12) which can act as a powerful irritant to animals. However, it gradually dimerizes to anemonin which is fairly harmless.

Another toxic plant glycoside is phloridzin (Fig. 7.13) which inhibits absorption of glucose from the intestine and from the kidney tubules, mimicking the symptoms of diabetes. It has also been reported to act as an uncoupler of oxidative phosphorylation at the final ADP phosphorylating step.

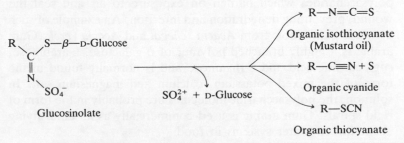

Fig. 7.11 Enzymic hydrolysis of glucosinolates.
R = variable organic moiety.

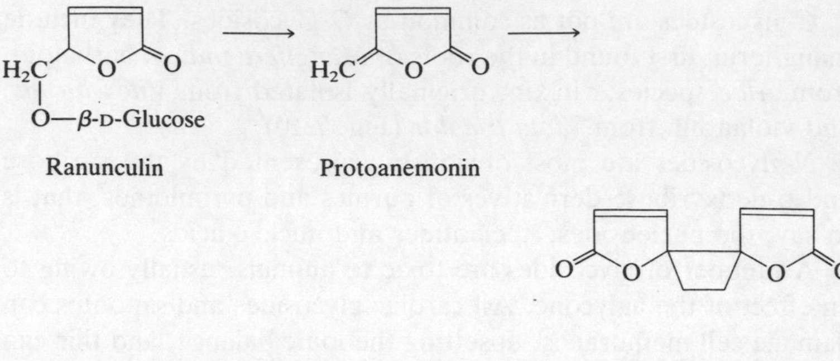

Ranunculin   Protoanemonin

Anemonin

Fig. 7.12 The conversion of ranunculin to protoanemonin and anemonin.

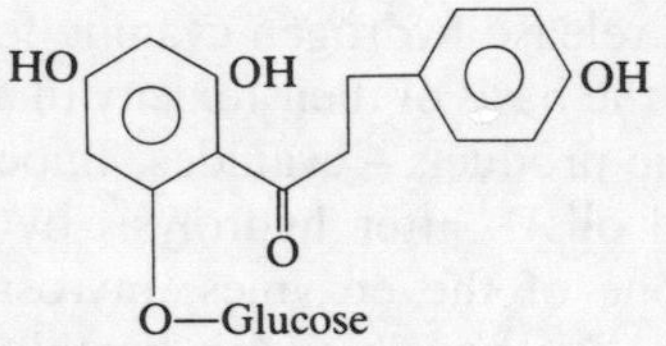

O—Glucose

Fig. 7.13 Phloridzin.

Much of the biological importance of glycosides still remains to be discovered but it is clear that they can act as deterrents to feeding (protecting plants from herbivores) and as insect attractants, both for feeding and egg laying. Elucidation of these functions may contribute to the development of 'natural' systems of pest control, reducing our dependence on synthetic pesticides.

7.4 Exudate gums

Many plants exude gums when they are wounded. These gums are polysaccharides which harden on exposure to air and seal the wound, preventing dehydration and infection. An example of such a gum is gum arabic from *Acacia senegal* and *Acacia verek*. Gum arabic is a highly branched polymer of D-galactose, L-arabinose, D-glucuronic acid and L-rhamnose and is normally found in the form of the mixed potassium, calcium and magnesium salt. In solution, the polysaccharide molecules are probably in the form of rigid spirals. Gum arabic is used commercially as an emulsifying agent for oil/water systems in food.

Gum ghatti is the exudate of *Anogeissus latifolia* which grows in India and Sri Lanka. It is a polymer of L-arabinose, D-galactose,

D-mannose, D-glucuronic acid and D-xylose and occurs naturally as the calcium salt.

Other gums of commercial significance are gum tragacanth from *Astragalus* spp., gum karaya from *Sterculia urens*, cholla gum from *Opuntia bulgida*, mesquite gum from *Prosopis juliflora* and khaya gums from *Khaya* spp.

7.5 Seaweed gums

Seaweed gums are cell wall components or reserve carbohydrates. Some of them have been put to commercial use. For example, alginic acid from brown algae is widely used in food because of its jellying and thickening properties. It consists of chains of L-mannuronic acid and D-guluronic acid. There are three types of region in these chains – a homogeneous L-mannuronic acid region, a homogeneous D-guluronic acid region and a heterogeneous region in which L-mannuronic acid and D-guluronic acid residues alternate. Linkage of residues is probably by β-(1→4)-linkages. The lengths and proportions of the different regions vary with the species of origin and these variations lead to different gross physical and chemical properties. Biosynthesis involves the GDP derivatives of the uronic acids.

Agar is used in food manufacture but perhaps its best known use is as a matrix for microbial cultures. It is produced by red algae, especially *Gelidium* and *Gracilaria* spp, and contains two polysaccharides, agarose and agaropectin. Agarose is a polymer of D-galactose, 3,6-anhydro-L-galactose and small amounts of D-xylose. Some of the D-galactose units are methylated at C-6. The principal structure consists of alternating segments of α-(1→3)-linked D-galactose residues and β-(1→4)-linked 3,6-anhydro-L-galactose. Agaropectin is very similar but contains D-glucuronic acid and small amounts of other sugars including sulphate esters.

Carrageenans are gums extracted from algae belonging to the Rhodophyceae. They are mixtures of polysaccharides largely made up of D-galactose residues with (1→3) and (1→4) linkages. Many of the galactose residues are sulphated.

7.6 Secondary products and chemosystematics

Often the somewhat restricted distribution of secondary products can contribute to the elucidation and understanding of phylogenetic relationships. For example, the cyclitol L-leucanthemitol,

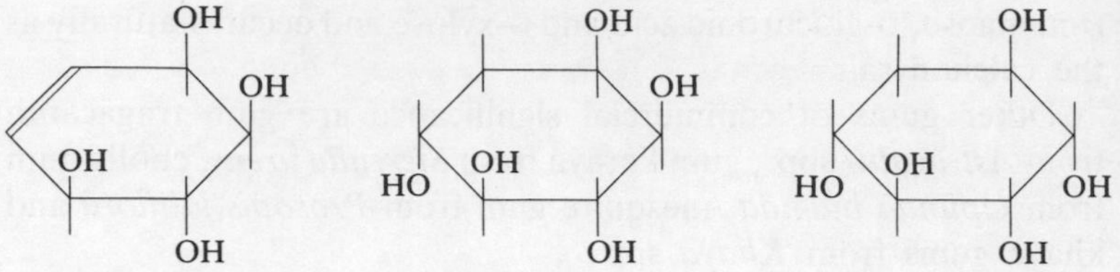

L-Leucanthemitol   L-Viburnitol   D-Quercitol

Fig. 7.14 Some cyclitols of importance in chemosystematics.

is found only in three species of *Chrysanthemum*, all of which belong to the Pyrethrum section of the genus. Another cyclitol, L-viburnitol, seems to be largely restricted to the Anthemidiae. Yet another cyclitol, D-quercitol, is present in all *Quercus* spp. but absent from the closely related *Fagus* and *Castanea* spp. (Fig. 7.14).

Glycosides can also be useful in chemosystematics. Amygdalin is a characteristic component of the Rosaceae. Quercetin-3-gentiobioside is found only in members of the Tribuleae tribe of the Zygophyllaceae, serving to confirm the view that this tribe should be treated as a separate family. Glucosinolates and cyanogenic glycosides have never been found in the same species. Other examples of the contribution of secondary products to chemosystematics can be found in the references cited at the end of the chapter but this is an area in which there is great scope for further research.

References

Conn, E. E. (ed.) (1981) Cyanogenic glycosides, in *The Biochemistry of Plants*, Vol 7 (P. K. Stumpf and E. E. Conn, eds.). Academic Press: New York and London.

Harborne, J. B. (ed.) (1972) *Phytochemical Ecology*. Academic Press: London and New York.

Harborne, J. B. (1977) *Introduction to Ecological Biochemistry*. Academic Press: London and New York.

Luckner, M. (1972) *Secondary Metabolism in Plants and Animals*. Chapman & Hall.

Northcote, D. H. (ed.) (1974) *Plant Biochemistry* Vol. 11 (Biochemistry Series One). Butterworths.

Runeckles, V. C. and Conn, E. E. (eds.) (1974) *Recent Advances in Phytochemistry*, Vol. 8. Academic Press: New York and London.

Swain, T. (ed.) (1963) *Chemical Plant Taxonomy*. Academic Press: London and New York.

Swain, T. (ed.) (1966) *Comparative Phytochemistry*. Academic Press: London and New York.

Swain, T. (ed.) (1973) *Chemistry in Evolution and Systematics*. Butterworths.

Vaughan, J. G. *et al.* (eds) (1976) *The Biology and Chemistry of the Cruciferae*. Academic Press: London and New York.

Vickery, Margaret L. and Vickery, B. (1981) *Secondary Plant Metabolism*. Macmillan.

8

Regulation of carbohydrate metabolism

8.1 General aspects of metabolic regulation

It is often possible to isolate enzymes and show that their activities may be controlled *in vitro* by changes in the concentration of compounds other than their substrates or products. The control may be demonstrated as an activation or an inhibition and may affect either the catalytic efficiency of the enzyme (measured by V_{max}) or the binding of the substrate to the active site (which would change the K_m). This kind of effect is often described as regulatory. However, any metabolic pathway can have only one rate-limiting step at which effective regulation can occur, even though it may include several enzymes which have been shown to exhibit regulatory effects as described above. Only the enzyme which catalyses the rate-limiting step can be truly regulatory with regard to a particular metabolic pathway but it is possible for the rate-limiting step to change as conditions change. Variations in substrate concentration, oxygen tension, hormonal balance, nutrition, etc. can cause such changes to occur. In this way, two or more enzymes may regulate one metabolic pathway, each acting under a different set of physiological conditions. Thus, the term 'regulatory' attached to an enzyme can rarely be regarded as an absolute description as it will often be true in a physiological sense only under certain specified conditions.

The term 'metabolic pathway' is best defined as an unbranched sequence of reactions converting one substance to another. This makes analysis of regulation fairly straightforward. Unfortunately, in traditional biochemistry the term has been used more loosely. For example, the glycolytic pathway (Emden–Meyerhof–Parnas pathway) involves various branching points starting with glucose-

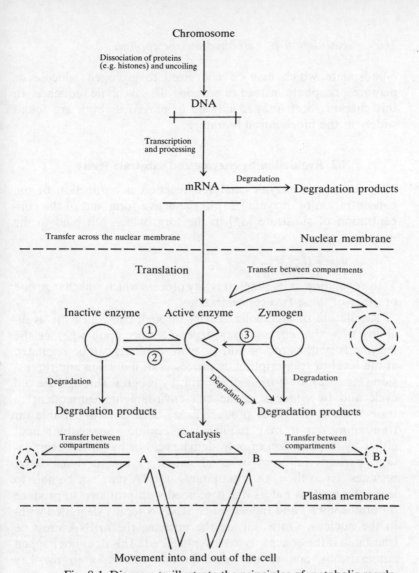

Fig. 8.1 Diagram to illustrate the principles of metabolic regulation. Each process illustrated has its own regulatory features and
can interact with the other processes; for example, the substrate
A might activate the inactive enzyme or induce transcription of
the DNA coding for the enzyme and hence its synthesis, thus
facilitating the conversion of A to B; a high concentration of
B might reverse these changes (feedback control) and so on.
(1) Activators, prosthetic groups or essential ions. Enzymic
     modification.
(2) Inactivators or processes removing prosthetic groups or
     essential ions. Enzymic modification.
(3) Proteases

6-phosphate which may be converted to glycogen, glucose or pentose phosphate instead of entering the glycolytic sequence. In this chapter, both usages may be employed as both are found widely in the biochemical literature.

8.2 Regulation by enzyme and substrate levels

The rate of an enzyme-catalysed reaction is a function of the concentration of enzyme $[E^*]$ in the active form and of the concentration of substrate $[S^*]$ in the form which can bind to the enzyme, i.e.:

$$\text{Rate} \propto [E^*][S^*]$$

Thus regulation at its simplest is any process which will change one or other of these two concentrations.

Regulation of metabolic activity through control of the availability of active enzyme may depend simply upon whether the enzyme is synthesized or not. Enzyme synthesis can be regulated at the level of transcription by processes of induction and repression (Fig. 8.2), by hormonal control, by progress through the cell cycle and by changes in the cell environment. Subsequent to transcription, the RNA produced may be in a form suitable for translation but it may require modification (processing) first, either by the addition of polyadenylic acid or by partial degradation, perhaps followed by combination of the surviving RNA residues. Even then, the translatable mRNA may not be able to leave the nucleus unless it is combined with proteins (to produce 'informosomes') and indeed much RNA is totally degraded within the nucleus. Once outside the nucleus, the mRNA must be translated if the enzyme is to be synthesized. This does not happen automatically and it may well be that this is often the key regulatory step. If synthesis of an enzyme is not closely controlled, selective degradation of the enzyme may be crucial in regulating its concentration.

Even after the enzyme has been synthesized it may not be available to catalyse reactions owing to physical or chemical compartmentation. Perhaps the most obvious example of physical compartmentation is the isolation of hydrolytic enzymes in lysosomes which prevents total cell autolysis occurring in healthy cells. Chemical compartmentation may involve zymogens as inactive precursors of enzymes, allosteric effects in which enzymes exist in interconvertible active and inactive forms, (Fig. 8.3) and enzymes

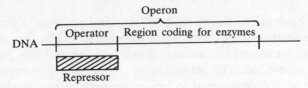

(a) Transcription of operon blocked by repressor protein

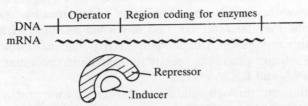

(b) Transcription of operon proceeds as repressor protein is removed by binding to inducer. The messenger RNA is translated and so the enzymes are induced.

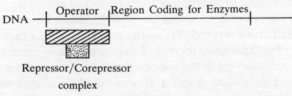

(c) Transcription of operon blocked by repressor/corepressor complex. In this case, the uncomplexed repressor protein cannot bind to the operator. Thus the corepressor represses transcription and enzyme synthesis.

Fig. 8.2 Diagram to show the operon mechanism of induction and repression of enzymes

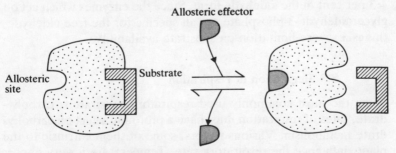

Fig. 8.3 Diagram to illustrate the conversion of an enzyme from an active to an inactive form by reversible combination with an allosteric effector

which are regulated by the binding of 'specifier' proteins. Zymogens are distinctive in that they function unidirectionally, i.e. the zymogen is hydrolysed to produce active enzyme and this process is not reversible. The activation of β-amylase in germinating barley may be considered to be an example of this kind of process. Two examples of allosterically controlled enzymes are described below in relation to the Pasteur effect and the regulation of starch biosynthesis in leaves. Regulation of enzymes by 'specifier' proteins may be rarer but one important example of an enzyme of this type is DNA-dependent RNA polymerase which requires the σ-factor protein to specify for binding to the initiator codons in DNA and RNA.

Strictly, the rate through a non-equilibrium enzymic reaction can only be limited by substrate concentration if the substrate concentration is near to or below the K_m value but this seems frequently to be the case. Limiting substrate concentrations can result from restricted production or from restricted availability as a result of compartmentation within the cell. Restricted availability may also result from interactions of the substrate with other cell components. For example, increased magnesium ion concentrations may cause lowering of the concentration of substrates such as citrate to which they bind. Substrates may bind to enzymes which are present in very large amounts and thus be rendered unavailable to other enzymes. Another restriction on substrate availability will be imposed if the substrate can exist in interconvertible forms and the internal milieu of the cell favours one with which the enzyme systems will not react. For instance, glyceraldehyde-3-phosphate at $37\,°C$ exists as 95.7 per cent in the hydrated form and 4.3 per cent in the aldehyde form. Since the enzymes which act on glyceraldehyde-3-phosphate are all specific for the free aldehyde, this is a severe limitation on substrate availability.

8.3 Regulation of respiration

Since the most commonly used respiratory substrate is carbohydrate, rates of respiration must have a profound effect on carbohydrate metabolism. Various factors, some of them extrinsic to the plant, influence the respiratory rate. Temperature is very important. For most temperate zone species, the optimum temperatures for respiration lie between 25 and $30\,°C$. (The optimum temperature referred to here is the highest temperature at which a steady state of respiration can be maintained for long periods of time.) The Q_{10} within the physiological range is 2 to 3. Interestingly, high rates of respiration are not always directly associated with high rates of starch breakdown. In potatoes, low temperatures favour the breakdown of starch at a rate faster than respiration can oxidize the products. This causes noticeable sweetening of the potatoes (§3.5).

Another factor controlling respiration is the ambient carbon dioxide concentration. Concentrations of carbon dioxide above about 5 per cent are generally considered to be inhibitory to respiration and 10 per cent carbon dioxide may be lethal. However, in some tissues, treatment with 45 to 70 per cent carbon dioxide over periods of 24 h or more has led to respiratory stimulation.

As might be expected, there is some evidence of response to substrate supply. Wheat leaves, for example, show increased respiration when supplied with sucrose. A factor which may influence substrate supply is the degree of hydration. Desiccation seems to move the starch–glucose balance towards glucose release.

Hormones may influence respiration profoundly. This is very marked in the fruit climacteric (Fig. 8.4). The onset of the climacteric is associated with the large-scale production of the gaseous growth regulator ethylene. Following this, tissues soften

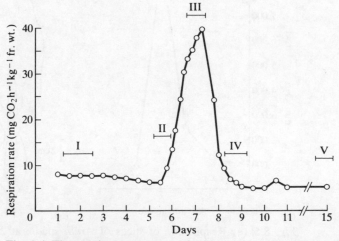

Fig. 8.4 The respiratory pattern of a honeydew melon *Cucumis melo* during the climacteric. The stages of ripening are indicated by the numerals: I, preclimacteric; II, onset of the climacteric; III, climacteric; IV, post-climacteric; V, fully ripe. (From H. C. Passam and M. C. Bird, 1978. *J. Exp. Bot.* **29**, 325.)

owing to the hydrolysis of cell wall pectins and breakdown of starch is accelerated. Initially, there is a slight drop in the rate of respiration but it rapidly rises to a peak (as much as 5 × the minimum value) before dropping back to the minimum. It is observed that there is an increase in the activity of phosphofructo-kinase which is generally regarded as the pacemaker of glycolysis.

A spectacular respiratory change is that which occurs in *Arum* spadix (Fig. 8.5). The very rapid respiration which occurs for a short time (1–2 h) in this organ late in flower development is associated with an increase in temperature of the organ to levels as high as 20 °C above ambient. The principal substrate for this is starch. Oxidation proceeds through glycolysis and the tricarboxylic acid cycle and the cyanide-insensitive respiratory system that is found in plants. The respiratory system is almost completely uncoupled and this accounts for the heat generated.

At the biochemical level, one of the best known effects on respiration is the Pasteur effect. At its simplest, it is the inhibition of glycolysis observed when cells are moved from anaerobic to

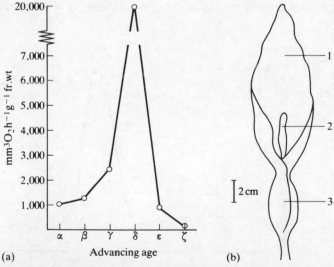

(a)   Advancing age   (b)

Fig. 8.5 (a) Respiration of slices of *Arum* spadix at 25 °C, at progressive stages of development, conventionally designated α to ξ; the entire sequence covers a few weeks. (From E. W. Simon, 1958. *J. Exp. Bot.* **10**, 125.)
(b) The inflorescence of *Arum maculatum* at thermogenesis; (1) spathe; (2) spadix; (3) enclosure containing the flowers.

aerobic conditions. The control system works through the enzyme phosphofructokinase (§4.2). For this enzyme, ATP is not only a co-substrate but also acts as an allosteric inhibitor. Since ADP and, to a much lesser extent, AMP are positive effectors overcoming ATP inhibition, the ratio ATP/ADP(AMP) controls the activity of the enzyme and hence the rate of glycolysis. Aerobic respiration usually raises ATP levels with the consequence that phosphofructokinase is inhibited. Conversely, if high rates of ATP utilization or anaerobiosis lower the ATP levels, the rate of glycolysis will increase.

8.4 Regulation of photorespiration

So far, our attention has been focused on respiration through glycolysis and the Krebs cycle. Such respiration may be referred to as 'dark', 'mitochondrial' or even 'normal' respiration. This respiration is saturated in leaves at 1–2 per cent oxygen in the atmosphere. Photorespiration is undetectable at such low oxygen levels and its rate increases with increasing oxygen tension all the way up to 100 per cent. High rates of photosynthesis are accompanied by high rates of photorespiration because the photorespiratory substrate, glycolate, is itself a product of photosynthesis (§4.7). Glycolate is formed from ribulose-1,5-bisphosphate by an oxygenation reaction catalysed by ribulose bisphosphate carboxy lase-oxygenase. This oxygenase reaction increases relative to the carboxylase activity as ambient temperature increases. Thus high temperatures favour photorespiration relative to photosynthesis. This can result in serious losses of fixed carbon from temperate crop plants. Many tropical crop plants have evolved a special form of leaf anatomy (Kranz anatomy) to minimize this problem (§1.2). The products of photorespiration are glyoxylate and hydrogen peroxide–the latter is decomposed by catalase to water and oxygen.

8.5 Regulation of starch degradation (§6.1)

Three possible modes of regulation of starch breakdown in leaves have been identified. Firstly, there is pH. Most enzymes involved in starch degradation have pH optima at or below pH 6.0. When photosynthesis is taking place in isolated chloroplasts in an ambient medium at pH 7.6, the stromal pH is 8.0. In the dark under the same conditions, the stromal pH is about 7.0. This pH drop should facilitate starch degradation.

Phosphate concentration may be another factor regulating starch degradation. It has been found that inorganic phosphate concentration in leaves is 30 to 50 per cent less in the light than in the dark and this may effectively limit phosphorylase activity.

Finally, light has been shown to activate an enzyme system which can reduce proteins. This might cause inactivation of some enzymes but it should be remembered that most enzymes seem to be more active in the reduced form and, of course, one of these more active enzymes is β-amylase (see below).

In germinating seeds, both enzyme activation and *de novo* synthesis play a part in initiation of starch degradation. β-Amylase in cereals is released from glutein, probably by the action of disulphide reductase but possibly also by the action of proteases. α-Amylase, on the other hand, is largely synthesized *de novo*, following the action of gibberellins either on the aleurone layers, as in barley, or on the scutellum as in maize. It is of some interest that there is a sequential appearance of enzyme activities in barley, pentosanase, glucanase and debranching enzymes increasing in activity before any increase in α-amylase activity. This may reflect the cell wall components which must be attacked before α-amylase can reach its substrate. In rice, the development of α-amylase activity is affected by light, the final activity being 3.5 times more in seeds germinated in the dark than in those exposed to light. In peas, not only is β-amylase released from a latent form but amylopectin α-(1→6)-glucosidase is activated, apparently by proteolytic activity as this effect can be simulated by trypsin.

8.6 Regulation of starch biosynthesis (§5.2)

In considerations of regulation of starch biosynthesis in leaves, attention has become centred on the enzyme ADP-glucose pyrophosphorylase. This enzyme is highly sensitive to activation by 3-phosphoglycerate, the primary photosynthetic carbon dioxide fixation product in C_3 plants and the secondary product generated by transcarboxylation in C_4 plants. The enzyme is also inhibited by inorganic phosphate. Thus, the enzyme will be highly active in the light as 3-phosphoglycerate concentrations build up and inorganic phosphate concentrations decrease. This in turn will lead to enhanced synthesis of starch or phytoglycogen from the precursor, ADP-glucose. It should be emphasized that the important factor in regulating ADP-glucose pyrophosphorylase is the ratio of the activator, 3-phosphoglycerate, to the inhibitor, inorganic phosphate, and not their absolute concentrations.

8.7 Miscellaneous enzymes showing regulatory properties related to carbohydrate metabolism

In some tissues, NAD^+-linked isocitrate dehydrogenase is probably the main controlling enzyme of the tricarboxylic acid cycle (see §4.5). The plant enzyme appears to be inhibited by high concentrations of inorganic anions and to be activated by citrate. At least one plant, *Brassica napus*, has an NAD^+-isocitrate dehydrogenase which is very sensitive to NADH inhibition. This raises the possibility of a control system acting through the NAD^+/NADH ratio and thereby reflecting the operation of the electron transport chain.

Fructose bisphosphatase is important in gluconeogenesis and if it is inhibited, gluconeogenesis will be suppressed and glycolysis will be stimulated (§4.3). It has been found that the alkaline fructose bisphosphatases from castor bean endosperm and wheat embryos are inhibited by AMP. Thus, under conditions where nearly all adenine nucleotides are fully phosphorylated, gluconeogenesis can occur, but if phosphorylation is impaired so that AMP accumulates, glycolysis is facilitated.

L-Glutamine-fructose-6-phosphate amidotransferase is the first enzyme in the pathway for the synthesis of uridine diphosphate-*N*-acetyl-D-glucosamine. It catalyses the following reaction:

$$\text{D-fructose-6-phosphate} + \text{L-glutamine}$$
$$\downarrow$$
$$\text{D-glucosamine-6-phosphate} + \text{L-glutamic acid}$$

This enzyme is competitively inhibited with regard to D-fructose-6-phosphate by the final product of the pathway it initiates. In this way, the cell concentration of uridine diphosphate-*N*-acetyl-D-glucosamine is kept fairly constant by feedback inhibition.

References

Denton, R. M. and Pogson, C. I. (1976) *Metabolic Regulation*. Chapman & Hall.

Ginsburg, V. and Robbins, P. (eds.) (1981) *Biology of Carbohydrates*, Vol. I. Wiley: New York.

Opik, H. (1968) *The Respiration of Higher Plants* (Studies in Biology, No. 120). Edward Arnold.

154   *Regulation of carbohydrate metabolism*

Preiss, J. and Kosuge, T. (1976) Regulation of enzyme activity in metabolic pathways, in *Plant Biochemistry* (3rd ed.) (J. Bonner and J. E. Varner, eds.). Academic Press: New York and London.

Richter, G. (1978) *Plant Metabolism*. Croom Helm: London; Georg Thieme: Stuttgart.

9

Techniques of carbohydrate analysis

9.1 Extraction of carbohydrates

As far as possible, plant carbohydrates are extracted by solubilization in aqueous solvents or in aprotic dipolar organic solvents such as dimethylsulphoxide. Care must be taken to minimize modification of the carbohydrates by endogenous enzymes or by the reagents used. Aqueous solutions of polysaccharides may be dialysed to remove inorganic salts and other low molecular weight impurities. Salts may also be removed by electrodialysis, by treatment with ion exchange resins or by gel filtration.

Carbohydrates may be obtained from aqueous solutions by freeze drying or, if they are polysaccharides, by precipitation with a miscible organic solvent such as ethanol or acetone. Fractional precipitation with these solvents may lead to the separation of different polysaccharides. Alternatively, fractional precipitation may be achieved by the use of metal ions or quaternary ammonium salts to form insoluble complexes with acidic polysaccharides, or by using reagents which co-ordinate with specific arrangements of hydroxyl groups.

Fractional precipitation may be sufficient to purify some polysaccharides completely but it is often necessary to use chromatographic methods to complete the purification. Chromatography on various forms of cellulose is usually effective. For charged polysaccharides, ion exchange chromatography on supports such as diethylaminoethyl (DEAE)-cellulose or DEAE-Sephadex can be used. DEAE-Sephadex combines the properties of an ion exchanger with those of a molecular sieve. Molecular sieve chromatography has been used for the separation of carbohydrates with molecular weights from 10^2–10^6 or more. Apart from Sephadex (a cross-linked dextran gel), porous silica beads may be used for this kind of separation. Such silica beads have the advantages of rigidity and chemical inertness. Molecular sieve chromatography may be used for molecular weight determination but it is limited by the difficulty in obtaining adequate standard materials for calibration of columns or thin layers.

9.2 Analysis of monosaccharides and oligosaccharides

Strictly speaking, complete characterization of a monosaccharide requires the isolation of at least one crystalline derivative in reasonable quantity. Often this may be possible following preparative thin layer or column chromatography using cellulose or Kieselguhr. However, where only milligram amounts are available, the application of a range of chromatographic methods is generally regarded as sufficient for an acceptable identification. The methods most frequently applied are paper partition chromatography, thin layer chromatography and gas–liquid chromatography though high pressure liquid chromatography is being used increasingly. Gas–liquid chromatography requires the preparation of volatile derivatives such as alditol acetates or *O*-trimethylsilyl (TMS) derivatives in which all the hydroxyl groups are masked. The main deficiency of chromatographic methods is that they do not permit a distinction to be made between the optical isomers of the D- and L-series.

Quantitative analysis of monosaccharides can be accomplished by the methods mentioned above, providing that calibration with mixtures of monosaccharides of known composition has been performed. In some cases, direct analysis of certain monosaccharides or monosaccharide groups may be carried out using selective colorimetric procedures or enzymic methods.

Ion exchange chromatography is the basis of the automated analysis of mono- and oligosaccharides and derived alditols. The aldoses are detected in the eluant with orcinol reagent. Both aldoses and alditols may be detected by periodate oxidation yielding formaldehyde which is estimated colorimetrically using pentane-2,4-dione.

Oligosaccharides may be analysed by paper or thin layer chromatography but complex mixtures will require the use of column chromatography as well. Neutral polysaccharides may be separated by partition chromatography on cellulose, gradient elution with aqueous ethanol from charcoal/celite, aqueous elution from cross-linked cation exchange resins or by molecular sieve chromatography on Sephadex. Acidic polysaccharides may be separated by elution with gradients of acetic or formic acid from anion exchange resins. DEAE-cellulose and DEAE-Sephadex are also used for charged oligosaccharides. Following isolation, most oligosaccharides will have to be further characterized by hydrolysis, methylation and periodate oxidation (see below).

The application of mass spectrometry to the effluent from gas–liquid chromatography of oligosaccharides permits valuable structural information to be obtained. For example, if the structural symmetry involved in alditol formation is avoided by reduction of disaccharides with sodium borodeuteride, mass spectra will permit a distinction to be made between linkages of (1→3) and (1→4) types. Mass spectrometry linked to gas–liquid chromatography is particularly good for the identification of methyl ethers (prepared for structural analysis – see below) after conversion to their alditol acetates.

9.3 Chemical methods for determination of polysaccharide structure

9.3.1 Introduction

Chemical analysis of polysaccharides depends upon determination of their structure. This, in turn, requires information on the nature and proportions of the monosaccharide units, the position and configuration of the glycosidic linkages, the sequence of monosaccharide units, the types of branching present (if any) and the location of substituents. Such information is usually obtained by degradation studies, mainly based on hydrolysis, often following structural modification, e.g. methylation. Oxidative degradation using periodate is an alternative to hydrolysis and yields different information. No single method is sufficient to define the structure of a polysaccharide and a wide range of studies may be required just to gain an approximate picture of the structure of one that is particularly complex (Fig. 9.1).

9.3.2 Acid hydrolysis

For polysaccharides, the first step in analysis is the determination of the monosaccharides released on complete hydrolysis. Usually treatment with N-mineral acid (preferably under nitrogen) at 100 °C for 4 h is used to achieve hydrolysis. It is important to

1. Total acid hydrolysis followed by chromatography
   – indicates what monosaccharides are present in the polymer.
2. Partial acid hydrolysis followed by chromatography
   – indicates sequence of monosaccharides.
3. Selective hydrolysis followed by chromatography
   – indicates sequence of monosaccharides and the nature of the linkages between them.
4. Full methylation followed by hydrolysis and chromatography
   – indicates the nature of the linkages between monosaccharide units.
5. Periodate oxidation followed by assay of periodate consumed and of formic acid, formaldehyde, carbon dioxide and ammonia produced. If oxidation is followed by reduction with sodium borohydride and acid hydrolysis, glycerol and polyhydric alcohol products are assayed
   – indicates the nature of the linkages between monosaccharide units and average chain length.
6. Polarimetric measurements and infrared spectra
   – indicate anomeric classification of linkages.
7. Determination of molecular weight and shape.

Fig. 9.1 The strategy of polysaccharide analysis

realize that such treatment may lead to some decomposition. For example, sialic acids, 3,6-anhydro-D- and L-galactose may be completely lost while D-fructose will be partially decomposed. The reducing sugars L-idose and L-gulose are largely converted to non-reducing 1,6-anhydro-derivatives. On the other hand, certain glycosidic linkages are hydrolysed with great difficulty and so a compromise must be reached between conditions giving complete hydrolysis and those giving minimal decomposition.

Having identified the component monosaccharides of the molecule, more information can be gained by partial hydrolysis and the isolation of component oligosaccharides. For example, the isolation of maltose in large amounts from the hydrolysis of starch provided strong evidence for the existence of α-D-$(1\rightarrow4)$-linkages in the parent molecule.

Many glycans contain various types of linkage which hydrolyse at differing rates. This may simplify analysis of a polysaccharide by ensuring that only some of the possible oligosaccharides survive partial hydrolysis. On the other hand, detection of the readily hydrolysed linkages will require a different depolymerization procedure or structural modification of the molecule to stabilize the weaker glycosidic bonds. In general, α-D-glycosidic linkages are more easily hydrolysed than β-D-linkages and bonds of the $(1\rightarrow6)$ type are generally more resistant to hydrolysis than others. Polysaccharides containing monosaccharide units in the furanose form, such as arabinose-containing polysaccharides, are hydrolysed under very mild conditions while polysaccharides containing pyranosides are much more stable. In contrast, some glycosidic linkages are unusually resistant to acid hydrolysis, e.g. those containing glycosiduronic acid linkages and hexosaminidic linkages.

Since monosaccharides undergo acid-catalysed glycosidation ('acid reversion'), there is the possibility that oligosaccharides isolated from acid hydrolysates are artefacts produced by this process. Acid reversion is favoured by high sugar concentrations and tends to produce oligosaccharides with $(1\rightarrow6')$ linkages from hexoses. It is usually assumed that an oligosaccharide obtained after acid hydrolysis is not artefactual if it is obtained in much higher yield than the same sugar isolated from the reversion of the component monosaccharide under comparable conditions. However, this does not allow for the possibility of reversion by intramolecular transglycosylation.

The progress of polysaccharide hydrolysis may be followed by various means including fall in viscosity, increase in reducing power, change in optical rotation of solutions, or chromatographic analysis of samples (usually by paper chromatography or by gel permeation chromatography).

A number of different acids have been used to cause hydrolysis. Sulphuric acid 0.5–1 M has been very commonly used for hydrolysis of pento- and hexopyranose oligo- and polysaccharides.

At the end of hydrolysis, the acid may be removed with a weak base anion exchange resin or by neutralization with barium carbonate or hydroxide followed by filtration to remove the barium sulphate and treatment of the filtrate with ion exchange resins to remove residual ions. Finally, the hydrolysate may be concentrated by evaporation under reduced pressure or by freeze drying.

Aqueous 3 per cent nitric acid is good for hydrolysing plant cell wall polysaccharides containing large numbers of pentose and hexuronic acid residues. Times from 4 to 12 h may be needed for nearly complete hydrolysis of glycopyranosyluronic acid linkages.

It must be remembered that long periods of hydrolysis may lead to some degradation of residues, e.g. 10 per cent of galacturonic acid residues may be eliminated (see also the beginning of this section).

   Other acids that may be used for hydrolysis include hydrochloric acid, though this destroys aldopentoses and hexuronic acids, and various organic acids (formic, acetic, oxalic and trifluoroacetic). Formic acid is useful for the hydrolysis of the otherwise insoluble polysaccharides and has been particularly applied to hexuronic acid containing polysaccharides and mannoglycans.

   Acetic acid hydrolysis (acetolysis) produces acetylated derivatives from which the parent molecules are obtained by catalytic transesterification with sodium or barium methoxide in methanol. Acetolysis may give products which differ from those obtained by mineral acid hydrolysis. For example, (1→6') linkages are susceptible to acetolysis but resistant to mineral acid while 6-deoxy-hexopyranosidic linkages show greater susceptibility to mineral acid. An artefact to watch for during acetolysis is the possible anomerization of glycosidic linkages.

   Where a polysaccharide contains reducing groups which are degraded by aqueous acids, e.g. 3,6-anhydrohexose units which are converted to hydroxymethylfurfural, methanolysis or mercaptolysis may be used in place of acids.

   Autohydrolysis may occur when aqueous 1 per cent solutions of ash-free glycans are heated. This causes the release of L-arabinofuranose and 6-deoxy-hexopyranose residues from the outer chains of polysaccharides leaving a hydrolysis-resistant core which may be separated by precipitation with ethanol or acetone.

9.3.3 Enzymic hydrolysis (see also Ch. 6)

Enzymic hydrolysis is increasingly used as an alternative to treatment with acid. If the specificity of the enzyme has been established, much useful structural information can be obtained from knowledge of which bonds are being broken and which resist hydrolysis. In general, carbohydrate hydrolases can be divided into *endo*-enzymes, attacking the polysaccharide chain at random though hydrolysing specific types of bond, and *exo*-enzymes which hydrolyse bonds in sequence from one end of the chain (usually the non-reducing end). *Exo*-enzymes will not continue hydrolysis beyond a branch point or other structural irregularity. β-Amylase is an example of an *exo*-enzyme while α-amylase is an example of an *endo*-enzyme (§6.1). β-Amylase is frequently used in polysaccharide analysis. The β-amylolysis limit is the degree of conversion of the treated polysaccharide into maltose, expressed as a percentage. This gives a measure of the average length of the outer chains and is a characteristic of various phytoglycogens and amylopectins. Pullulanase (Fig. 9.2) may be the most useful *endo*-enzyme for structural analysis. This debranching enzyme is isolated from *Aerobacter aerogenes* and quantitatively hydrolyses pullulan to maltotriose (cf. debranching enzymes, §6.1.6). Pullulanase cannot on its own hydrolyse all the branch linkages in amylopectin and phytoglycogen but, when combined with high concentrations of β-amylase, will convert these substrates completely to maltose and glucose. The glucose arises from chains containing an odd number of glucose residues. Thus, measurement of the glucose and maltose produced permits assay of the average unit chain length of amylopectin and phytoglycogen.

Treatment of phytoglycogen or amylopectin successively with an *exo*-enzyme and then with a debranching enzyme permits determination of the degree of multiple branching. Enzymes which have been used include the *exo*-enzymes phosphorylase and β-amylase and the debranching enzymes amylo-1,6-glucosidase, pullulanase and bacterial isoamylase.

The range of enzymes potentially available for selective hydrolysis of polysaccharides is now very wide as a result of the

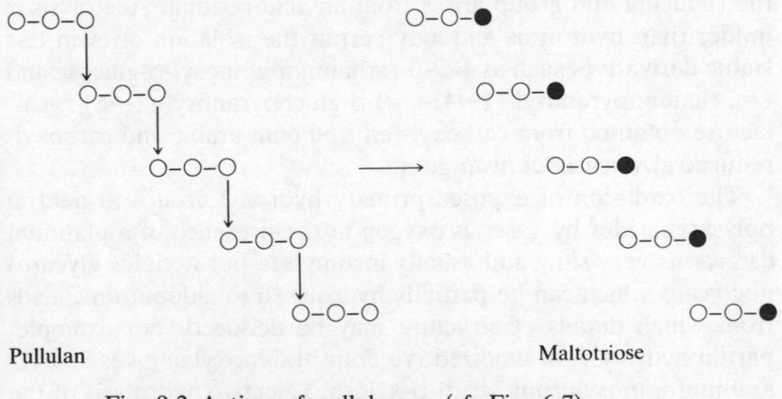

Pullulan   Maltotriose

Fig. 9.2 Action of pullulanase (cf. Fig. 6.7)
↓ = α-(1→6)-linkage
○ = α-(1→4)-linked non-reducing D-glucosyl residue
● = α-(1→4)-linked reducing D-glucosyl residue

possibilities for induction of enzymes in micro-organisms following exposure to simple glycosides of the required configuration. For example, methyl α-D-glucopyranoside may be used to induce α-D-glucosidase.

Not all the enzymes used for polysaccharide analysis are glycosidases. Esterases, sulphatases, peptidases and proteases may be employed to identify substituents or to liberate polysaccharides from linkage to peptides or proteins.

Like acid hydrolysis, enzymic hydrolysis is reversible and the possibility of the production of new oligosaccharides by transglycosylation must never be forgotten.

9.3.4 Hydrolytic degradation of reduced or oxidized polysaccharides

Glycuronoglycans are difficult to hydrolyse in their native state without destruction of the component monosaccharides. However, if the carboxyl groups are reduced to primary alcohol groups, complete or partial hydrolysis may be achieved without their destruction. Further, the oligosaccharides obtained may differ from those produced by partial hydrolysis of the original compound. Acid hydrolysis of glycuronoglycan will produce aldobiuronic acids but oligosaccharides containing neutral monosaccharide residues linked glycosidically to glycuronic acid residues will not be found. However, if the glycuronoglycan is reduced first, acid hydrolysis can yield oligosaccharides in which the reducing end group arises from an acid residue. Acetolysis is milder than hydrolysis and may permit the isolation of even less stable derivatives such as 4-*O*-α-L-rhamnopyranosyl-D-glucose and *O*-L-rhamnopyranosyl-(1→4)-*O*-β-D-glucopyranosyl-(1→6)-D-galactose obtained from carboxyl-reduced gum arabic and carboxyl-reduced *Araucaria bidwilli* gum.

The oxidation of exposed primary hydroxyl groups in neutral polysaccharides by gaseous oxygen in the presence of a platinum catalyst is very slow and usually incomplete but it yields glycuronoglycans which can be partially hydrolysed to aldobiuronic acids from which details of structure may be deduced. For example, partial hydrolysis of oxidized rye flour arabinoxylan gives 3-*O*-(L-arabinofuranosyluronic acid)-D-xylose. Selective hydrolysis of the unoxidized polysaccharide leaves a degraded xylan after removal of the L-arabinofuranose residues. Thus, it is likely that the L-arabinofuranose units are individually joined to the xylan core.

9.3.5 Degradation of methylated polysaccharides

Degradation of methylated polysaccharides is one of the main ways of analysing linkages in polysaccharides (Figs. 9.3 and 9.4). All the free hydroxyl groups in the polysaccharide of interest are methylated and then the glycosidic linkages are hydrolysed to give O-methyl monosaccharides or their derivatives. Analysis of the types of O-methyl monosaccharides and the amounts released enables conclusions to be reached regarding the relative proportions of non-reducing and reducing end groups, the nature of the main linkage types and the types of interchain linkages at branch points.

Haworth developed the technique of methylation of polysaccharides using dimethyl sulphate and sodium or potassium hydroxide in a nitrogen atmosphere at 10–55°C. This procedure has the disadvantage that several treatments with the reagents are often necessary. However, there is the advantage that, unlike other methods, degradation of acidic glycans is minimal. Variations on this method include the use of tetrahydrofuran as the solvent for dimethyl sulphate and powdered sodium hydroxide (permitting more extensive methylation and also combined methylation and de-acetylation of acetylated glycans), the use of dimethylsulphoxide as the solvent for dimethyl sulphate and sodium hydroxide, and the use of N,N-dimethylformamide or dimethylsulphoxide as solvents for dimethyl sulphate and barium hydroxide or barium oxide.

Purdie developed an alternative method using aqueous methyl iodide and silver oxide. This method cannot be applied to unmethylated polysaccharides but can complete the methylation of partially methylated glycans and of carboxyl groups in methylated acid glycans. The use of N,N-dimethylformamide as the solvent makes the method more efficient.

Hakomori modified Purdie's method to permit complete and rapid methylation of neutral and acid glycans dissolved in dimethyl sulphoxide using sodium methylsulphinyl methanide (sodium dimsyl) and methyl iodide as the reagents. This is currently the method of choice. Another modification of methylation by the use of methyl iodide is to heat it with thallium salts of acid glycans and a little anhydrous methanol; in this way acid glycans are rapidly esterified.

Once complete methylation of the polysaccharide has been accomplished, depolymerization of the resultant molecule usually takes place without much de-etherification. The method of degradation most commonly applied is to heat a 1–2 per cent solution of the methylated polysaccharide in 1–6 per cent methanolic hydrogen chloride under reflux on a boiling water bath until the optical rotation of the solution reaches a constant value. The solution is cooled and neutralized with silver carbonate or a weak base anion exchange resin, filtered and the filtrate concentrated under reduced pressure. Quantitative analysis of the methanolysate is then carried out, generally using chromatographic methods as described earlier in this chapter in §9.2.

The process of methylation and its usefulness in structural analysis are illustrated in Fig. 9.3. It should be noted, however, that some methylated sugars do not precisely define the ring size of the original sugars and their sites of substitution. For example, 2,3,6-tri-O-methyl-D-glucose (Fig. 9.4) could come from either a 4-O-substituted D-glucofuranose residue or a 5-O-substituted D-glucofuranose residue. Independent evidence is needed to distinguish between these structural possibilities.

If all the methylated sugars can be separated, the method described is limited mainly by difficulty in obtaining complete methylation and by the small degree of demethylation that may accompany hydrolysis. In principle, the methylation method permits determination of the sugar units in a polysaccharide and their mode of linkage. However, a problem may arise in relation to the presence or absence of branching. A small amount of di-O-methyl-D-glucose may arise from a branching point or from incomplete methylation. To distinguish between these possibilities, one must compare the value obtained for the average chain length using methylation end-group assay with the value for degree of polymerization obtained from the number-average molecular weight of the methylated polysaccharide. For instance, methylation end-group assay may give a chain length of n units from calculation of the reciprocal of the proportion of tetra-O-methyl-D-glucose from non-reducing end groups as a fraction of the total number of residues of this sugar. This value may be compared with a degree of polymerization value of n, in which case there is no branch point, or with a degree of polymerization value of $2n$, in which case there is a single branch point.

9.3.6 Periodate oxidation and Smith degradation

Where the main structural features of a polysaccharide are known, periodate oxidation causing glycol cleavage may provide further information about the types of glycosidic linkages present (Fig. 9.5). This technique may also provide valuable quantitative

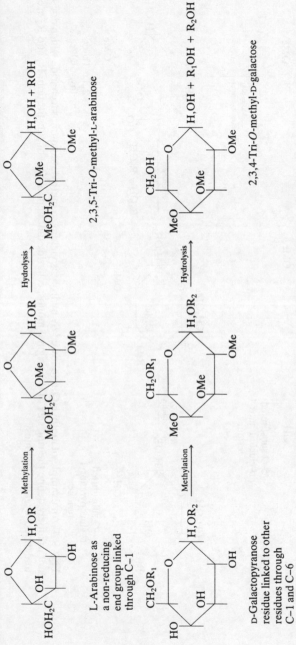

Fig. 9.3 Examples of *O*-methyl monosaccharides obtained by hydrolysis of fully methylated glycosides. Each of these methylated derivatives uniquely defines the ring size of the original monosaccharide and its linkage sites.

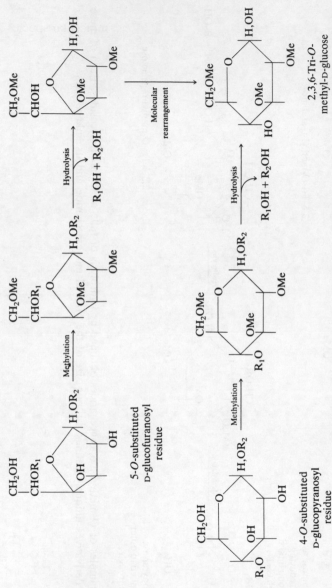

Fig. 9.4 An example of methylation followed by hydrolysis yielding a methylated monosaccharide which does not uniquely define the ring size of the original monosaccharide unit and its sites of substitution. R_1 and R_2 are undefined organic residues.

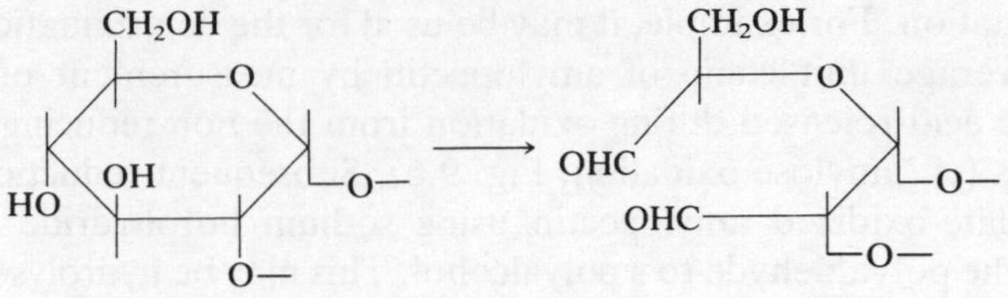

1 → 2 linkage

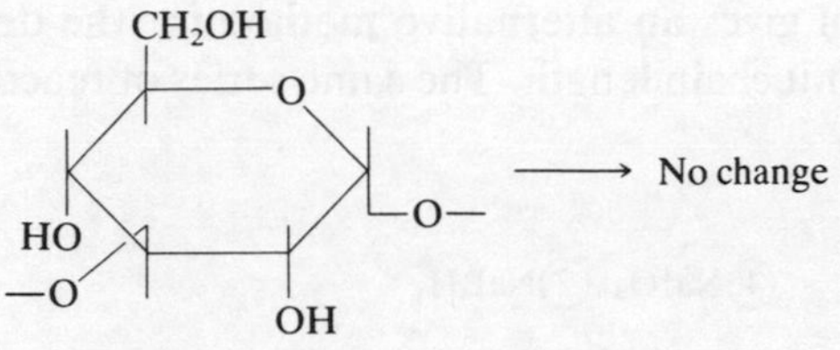

1 → 3 linkage

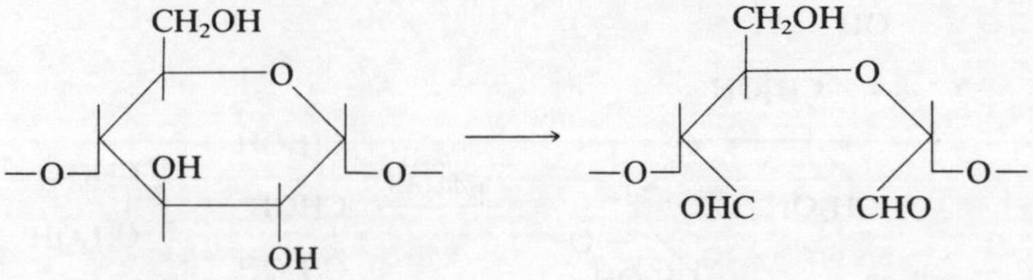

1 → 4 linkage

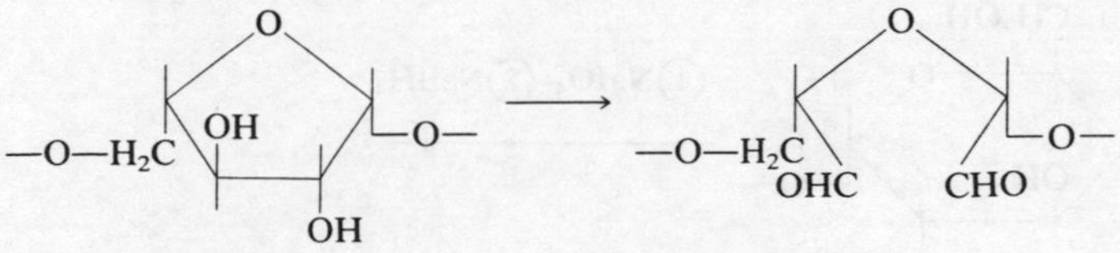

1 → 5 linkage

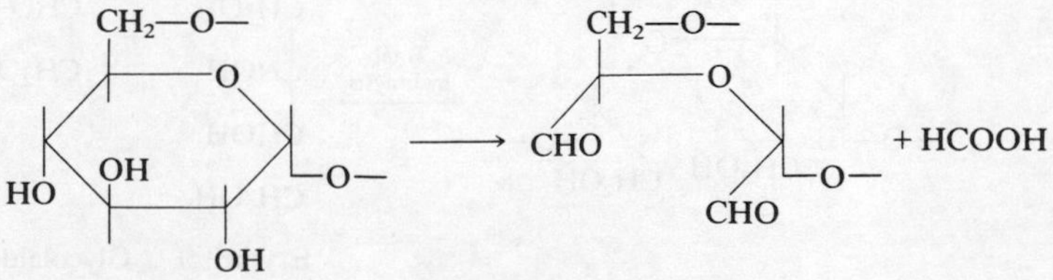

1 → 6 linkage

Fig. 9.5 The action of periodate on glucosyl residues with various linkages.

information. For example, it may be used for the determination of the average unit chain of amylopectin by measurement of the formic acid released during oxidation from the non-reducing end groups (cf. amylose oxidation, Fig. 9.6). Subsequent reduction of periodate-oxidized amylopectin using sodium borohydride converts the polyaldehyde to a polyalcohol. This may be hydrolysed to give glycolaldehyde, erythritol and glycerol. Since glycerol arises only from non-reducing end groups, measurement of amounts of glycerol and erythritol gives an alternative method for the determination of average unit chain length. The same series of reactions

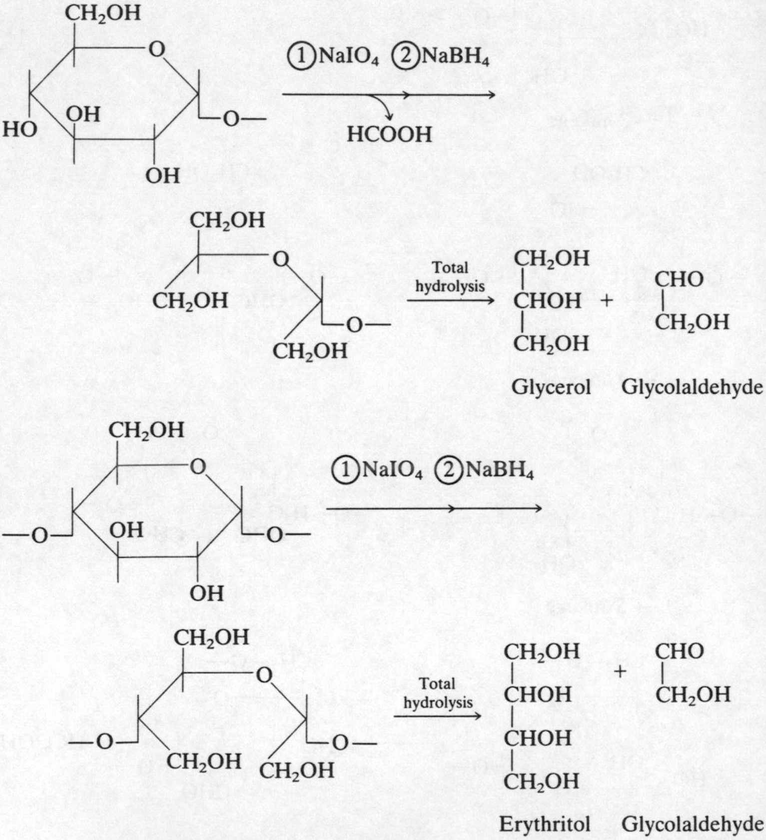

Fig. 9.6 Degradation of periodate oxidized amylose by total hydrolysis following sodium borohydride reduction yields glycerol, erythritol and glycolaldehyde. The formic acid and glycerol come only from non-reducing end groups as shown above.

releases monosaccharides from the residues which were not attacked by periodate.

Smith degradation is a useful modification of the above set of reactions. The polyalcohol produced by reduction with sodium borohydride is partially hydrolysed with dilute mineral acid at room temperature; this leads to selective hydrolysis of acyclic acetal linkages with the release of glycosides of polyhydric alcohols (Fig. 9.7). If a polysaccharide contains a number of adjacent

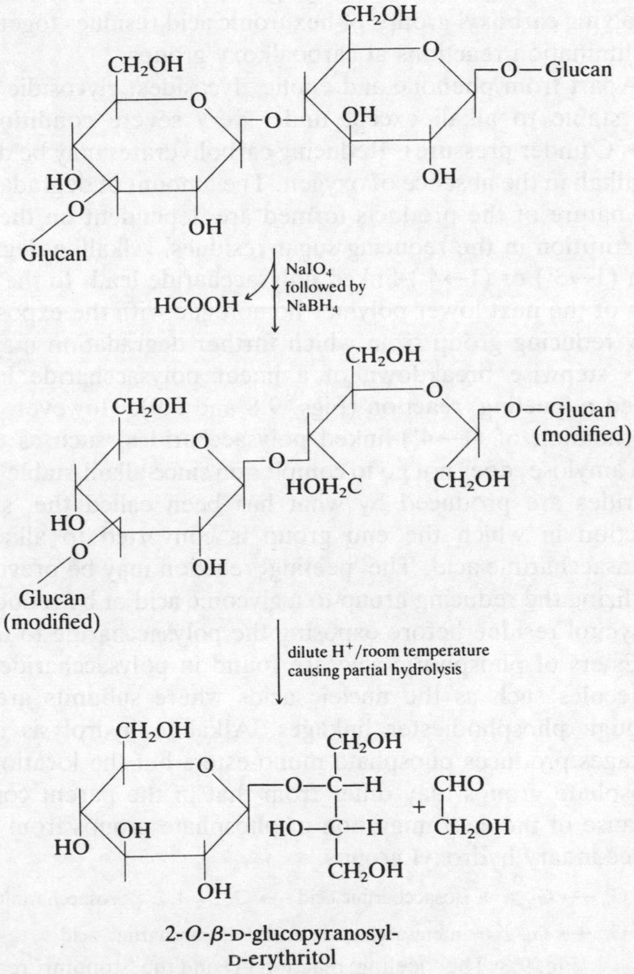

2-*O*-β-D-glucopyranosyl-D-erythritol

Fig. 9.7 Smith degradation of oat glucan showing the modification of the repeating unit.

non-oxidizable sugar residues, Smith degradation gives a degraded polysaccharide. This is what happens with larch arabinolactans.

9.3.7 Reactions with alkali

Many polysaccharides are extracted from plants with alkali and hence it is essential to know what changes can occur to carbohydrates under alkaline conditions. There are three principal effects – degradations starting at the reducing group, hydrolysis of esters involving sugar hydroxyl groups and hydrolysis of esters involving carboxyl groups of hexuronic acid residues together with β-elimination reactions at carboalkoxy groups.

Apart from phenolic and enolic glycosides, glycosidic linkages are stable to alkali except under very severe conditions (e.g. 170 °C under pressure). Reducing carbohydrates may be degraded by alkali in the absence of oxygen. The amount of degradation and the nature of the products formed are dependent on the sites of substitution in the reducing sugar residues. Alkaline degradation of a $(1 \rightarrow 3')$ or $(1 \rightarrow 4')$-linked polysaccharide leads to the production of the next lower polymer homologue with the exposure of a new reducing group from which further degradation may occur. This stepwise breakdown of a linear polysaccharide has been called a 'peeling' reaction (Figs. 9.8 and 9.9). However, alkaline degradation of $(1 \rightarrow 4')$-linked polysaccharides, such as cellulose and amylose, does not go to completion since alkali-stable polysaccharides are produced by what has been called the 'stopping' reaction in which the end group is converted to alkali-stable metasaccharinic acid. The 'peeling' reaction may be prevented by oxidizing the reducing group to a glyconic acid or by reducing it to a glycitol residue before exposing the polysaccharide to alkali.

Esters of phosphoric acid are found in polysaccharide macromolecules such as the nucleic acids where subunits are joined through phosphodiester linkages. Alkaline hydrolysis of these linkages produces phosphate mono-esters but the location of the phosphate groups may differ from that in the parent compound because of the easy migration of phosphate groups from primary to secondary hydroxyl groups.

(1) $G_n \longrightarrow G_{n-1}$ + isosaccharinic acid $\longrightarrow G_{n-2}$ + 2 × isosaccharinic acid $\longrightarrow$

(2) $G_n \longrightarrow G_{n-2}-$ metasaccharinic acid + isosaccharinic acid

> Fig. 9.8 The 'peeling' reaction (1) and the 'stopping' reaction (2) in alkaline degradation of $1 \rightarrow 4$ linked glucans.
> G = D-glucose residue

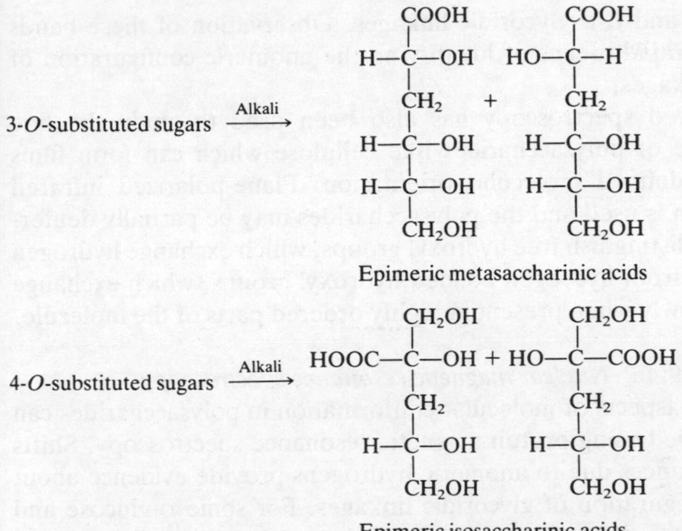

3-*O*-substituted sugars $\xrightarrow{\text{Alkali}}$

$$
\begin{array}{cc}
\text{COOH} & \text{COOH} \\
| & | \\
\text{H—C—OH} & \text{HO—C—H} \\
| & | \\
\text{CH}_2 \quad + & \text{CH}_2 \\
| & | \\
\text{H—C—OH} & \text{H—C—OH} \\
| & | \\
\text{H—C—OH} & \text{H—C—OH} \\
| & | \\
\text{CH}_2\text{OH} & \text{CH}_2\text{OH}
\end{array}
$$

Epimeric metasaccharinic acids

4-*O*-substituted sugars $\xrightarrow{\text{Alkali}}$

$$
\begin{array}{cc}
\text{CH}_2\text{OH} & \text{CH}_2\text{OH} \\
| & | \\
\text{HOOC—C—OH} \; + & \text{HO—C—COOH} \\
| & | \\
\text{CH}_2 & \text{CH}_2 \\
| & | \\
\text{H—C—OH} & \text{H—C—OH} \\
| & | \\
\text{CH}_2\text{OH} & \text{CH}_2\text{OH}
\end{array}
$$

Epimeric isosaccharinic acids

Fig. 9.9 Products of alkaline degradation of 3-*O*-substituted and 4-*O*-substituted sugars.

Esters of hexuronic acids occur in the methyl D-galacturonate residues of pectins. These esters are hydrolysed and saponified on treatment with alkali but a base-catalysed β-elimination reaction occurs as well and leads to the cleavage of glycosidic linkages.

9.3.8 Immunochemical reactions
Most polysaccharides are antigenic and can be used to produce antibodies of various specificities. These antibodies can be used to identify the presence of antigenic groups with which they interact causing precipitation. The amount of precipitate gives a measure of the quantity of antigen present.

9.4 Physical methods for determination of polysaccharide structure

9.4.1 Infrared spectroscopy
Using infrared spectroscopy, characteristic group frequencies can be recognized. Important groups which can be recognized in this way include carbonyl groups, acetamido groups and sulphate esters. In a number of homopolysaccharides such as glucans, absorption bands at $844 \pm 8\,\text{cm}^{-1}$ and $891 \pm 7\,\text{cm}^{-1}$ are associated

172   *Techniques of carbohydrate analysis*

with α- and β-D-glycosidic linkages. Observation of these bands gives a rapid means of identifying the anomeric configuration of such linkages.

Infrared spectroscopy has also been used to study the fine structure of polysaccharides like cellulose which can form films with a defined molecular orientation. Plane-polarized infrared radiation is used and the polysaccharides may be partially deuterated to distinguish free hydroxyl groups, which exchange hydrogen readily, from hydrogen bonded hydroxyl groups, which exchange quite slowly when present in highly ordered parts of the molecule.

9.4.2 Nuclear magnetic resonance spectroscopy

Various aspects of molecular conformation in polysaccharides can be clarified using proton magnetic resonance spectroscopy. Shifts of resonances due to anomeric hydrogens provide evidence about the configuration of glycosidic linkages. For some D-glucose and D-galactose derivatives, 1→4 linkages may be distinguished from 1→2 and 1→6 linkages. The positions of methyl substitution in ethers of D-glucopyranose and D-galactopyranose have been ascertained by reference to the chemical shifts of methoxyl signals in their perdeuteric-methylated methyl glycosides. These are only a few of the possibilities and it is certain that this technique can accomplish much more.

9.4.3 X-ray diffraction

The use of X-ray diffraction is restricted by the relatively small number of X-ray reflections given by polysaccharides, even when they are in the form of highly orientated fibres. However, X-ray diffraction by polysaccharide fibres does give information on the fibre repeat distance and an indication of the nature of the chain symmetry.

9.4.4 Molecular size and shape determination

Most polysaccharide preparations contain a mixture of molecules of various sizes and measurements of molecular weight give an average which depends upon the method used. The average obtained may be a number-average, biased towards the small molecules, or a weight-average, biased towards the larger molecules. The differences between number-average and weight-average provide a measure of the polydispersity of the polysaccharide. A number-average molecular weight is calculated from an equation of the type, $\bar{M}_n = \Sigma c_i \div \Sigma(c_i/M_i)$, where $\bar{M}_n$ is the number-average molecular weight, c_i is the concentration of the ith molecular species in g/cm^3 and M_i is the molecular weight of the ith molecular species. On the other hand, a weight-average molecular weight is calculated from an equation of the type, $\bar{M}_w = \Sigma c_i M_i \div \Sigma c_i$, where $\bar{M}_w$ is the weight average molecular weight and the others are as previously defined.

The method of number-average molecular weight determination to be used depends upon the molecular weight range of the polysaccharide. In the range 2,000 to 20,000, the method used is measurement of differences in vapour pressure between a solution of the carbohydrate and pure solvent at constant temperature (isothermal distillation) or measurement of differences between the boiling points of solution and solvent (ebulliometry). The problem with these methods is that they decrease in sensitivity as the molecular size of the solute increases. In the range 20,000 to 500,000, measurement of osmotic pressure is the only method which can be used to obtain acceptable number-average weights. Chemical methods for end-group assay have been used but they can be very sensitive to impurities, stoicheiometry of reactions with large molecules is often uncertain and not all end groups are necessarily identical in a population of molecules isolated from a natural source.

Weight-average molecular weights may be determined by measuring the difference in light scattering by a solution of polysaccharide and by the pure solvent. In addition, the dissymmetry of the scattered light may be used to estimate the molecular shape.

Ultracentrifugation may be used to give a molecular weight average but this average depends upon molecular shape. Sedimentation velocity is measured during centrifugation by following changes in the refractive index gradient of the polysaccharide solution. If the diffusion coefficient of the polysaccharide is known, the molecular weight can be estimated. Comparison of the observed hydrodynamic behaviour with that calculated for molecular models permits molecular shape to be deduced.

References

Aspinall, G. O. (1972) Degradation of polysaccharides, in *Weissberger's Techniques of Organic Chemistry*, Vol. IV, Elucidation of Structures (2nd edn.) (K. W. Bentley and G. W. Kirby, eds.), pp. 379–450. Wiley: New York.

174 Techniques of carbohydrate analysis

Aspinall, G. O. and Stephen, A. M. (1976) Polysaccharide methodology and plant polysaccharides, in *MTP International Review of Science*, *Carbohydrates* (Organic Chemistry Series Two, Vol. 7) (Consultant ed. D. H. Hey; Volume ed. G. O. Aspinall). Butterworths: London; University Park Press: Baltimore.

Aspinall, G. O. (1970) *Polysaccharides*. Pergamon.

Aspinall, G. O. (ed.) (1982) The Polysaccharides, Vol. 1, Academic Press.

Percival, E. G. V. (1962) *Structural Carbohydrate Chemistry* (2nd edn. revised). J. Garnett Miller.

Phelps, C. F. (1972) *Polysaccharides* (Oxford Biology Readers No. 27). Oxford University Press.

Pigman, W. and Horton, D. (eds.) (1970) *The Carbohydrates, Chemistry and Biochemistry*. Academic Press: New York.

Rees, D. A. (1977) *Polysaccharide Shapes. Outline Studies in Biology*. Chapman & Hall.

Whistler, R. L. (ed.) (1962–   ) *Methods in Carbohydrate Chemistry*. Academic Press: New York.

Index

féria, verde, missa à escolha. / **Leituras:** 1,24 – 2,3; Lc 6,6-11. / **Santos:** Alexan-, Jacinto, Severino.

do Veterinário e Dia do Administra- de Empresas

humа lei humanа deve nos impedir de izarmos obras de misericórdia.

emes muito o sofrimento, se ele não é a agradável para ti, não faças mal a nin- , nem abertamente, nem em segredo.

Udanavargа

* SET * SEG

EM. COMUM
/ + 113

9

ente